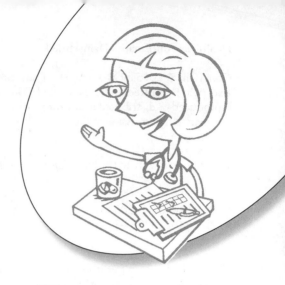

Healthcare Informatics
DeMYSTiFieD

D0573375

Jim Keogh, MSN, RN-BC

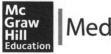 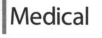

Mc Graw Hill Education | Medical

New York   Chicago   San Francisco   Athens   London   Madrid
Mexico City   Milan   New Delhi   Singapore   Sydney   Toronto

Healthcare Informatics Demystified

1 2 3 4 5 6 7 8 9 0   DOC/DOC   19 18 17 16 15 14

ISBN 978-0-07-182053-0
MHID 0-07-182053-1

This book was set in Berling by Cenveo® Publisher Services.
The editors were Andrew Moyer and Christina M. Thomas.
The production supervisor was Richard Ruzycka.
Project management was provided by Kritika Kaushik, Cenveo Publisher Services.
RR Donnelley was the printer and binder.

Notice

Medicine is an ever-changing science. As new research and clinical experience broaden our knowledge, changes in treatment and drug therapy are required. The authors and the publisher of this work have checked with sources believed to be reliable in their efforts to provide information that is complete and generally in accord with the standard accepted at the time of publication. However, in view of the possibility of human error or changes in medical sciences, neither the editors nor the publisher nor any other party who has been involved in the preparation or publication of this work warrants that the information contained herein is in every respect accurate or complete, and they disclaim all responsibility for any errors or omissions or for the results obtained from use of the information contained in this work. Readers are encouraged to confirm the information contained herein with other sources. For example and in particular, readers are advised to check the product information sheet included in the package of each drug they plan to administer to be certain that the information contained in this work is accurate and that changes have not been made in the recommended dose or in the contraindications for administration. This recommendation is of particular importance in connection with new or infrequently used drugs.

Library of Congress Cataloging-in-Publication Data

Keogh, James Edward, 1948- author.
    Healthcare informatics demystified / Jim Keogh.
        p. ; cm.
    Includes index.
    ISBN 978-0-07-182053-0 (paperback)—ISBN 0-07-182053-1 (paperback)
    I. Title.
    [DNLM: 1. Nursing Informatics. WY 26.5]
    RT50.5
    610.730285—dc23
                             2014004141

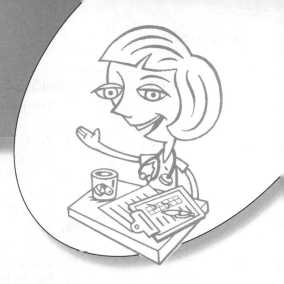

Contents

Introduction

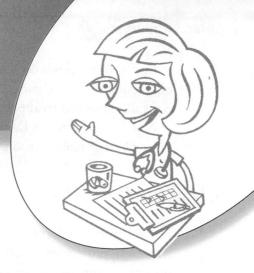

Computers and computer applications are the backbone of today's healthcare. A patient who does not feel right seeks medical help by asking the healthcare provider to diagnose the problem and prescribe treatment that will return the patient to activities of daily living. The healthcare provider uses a computer application to review the patient's medical history that includes recent visits, diagnoses, medication, and treatments.

If the patient needs to be admitted to the hospital, computer applications are used to collect admitting information. The computerized physician order entry (CPOE) system is used by practitioners to write medical orders. The order management system processes orders and displays results of orders entered by practitioners and nurses. The electronic medication administration record (eMAR) system is used by nurses to identify medications to administer to the patient and record when the medications are given. The physician documentation system enables practitioners to electronically document the practitioner's interactions with the patient. The electronic medical record (EMR) system is the patient's chart that is used by the patient's medical team to record electronically all information about the patient's stay.

All clinical computer applications are implemented by a team of clinical and management information systems (MIS) specialists typically led by a nurse who specializes in nursing informatics. The nursing informatics specialists interact with the clinical staff and administrater to identify clinical needs and then fulfill those needs working with MIS and third-party vendors.

In *Nursing Informatics Demystified*, you will learn the nursing informatics interventions and techniques used to apply computer technology to assist clinicians diagnose and treat patients.

Nursing Informatics Demystified contains 10 chapters, each providing a description of major nursing informatics interventions and techniques.

A Look Inside

Because nursing informatics can be challenging for beginners, this book has been written to provide an organized outline approach to learning about major components of nursing informatics and the part nurses can play in the MIS process. The following paragraphs provide a thumbnail description of each chapter.

Chapter 1 Nursing Informatics

Nursing informatics is the area of nursing that combines nursing, information, and computer sciences to manage information required for use in the nursing practice. The American Nurses Association (ANA) defines nursing informatics as a specialty that integrates nursing science, computer science, and information science to manage and communicate data, information, knowledge, and wisdom in nursing practice. The ANA recognized nursing informatics as a specialty in 1992.

The goal of nursing informatics is to support decision making of patients, practitioners, and nurses through the use of structured information and technology with the goals of reducing errors, improving communication, and promoting the use of evidence-based practice in all specialties of nursing.

At times there can be a blur between the role of MIS and the role of nursing informatics because both focus on providing computerization of clinical workflows. MIS is responsible for applications, computer hardware, networking, security, and everything involved in providing MIS to the entire healthcare facility.

Nursing informatics focuses on clinical applications, primarily analyzing clinical workflows, assessing the capabilities of clinical applications, and integrating clinical application into the healthcare facility's clinical workflow. In addition, the nursing clinical informatics specialist assists in developing policies and procedures related to clinical workflows and joins committees on meaningful use and core measurement, which are used by regulatory bodies to measure the performance of the healthcare facility.

Nursing informatics is frequently part of the MIS organization and is staffed by nurses who have had substantial clinical experiences both as first-line healthcare providers and in administration. Furthermore, the nursing informatics specialist has the necessary MIS training in clinical systems analysis, clinical database analysis, and clinical project management. The combination of MIS and clinical skills places the nursing informatics specialist in a unique position to improve clinical workflows through computer automation.

Chapter 2 Clinical Systems Analysis

A system is a group of interrelated components that function together to achieve a desired result. Simply said, a system is a way of doing something. It can be a manual process such as taking a telephone order from a practitioner. It can be an electronic process such as a CPOE. Or it can be a combination of manual and electronic processes such as taking a telephone order that is processed by the pharmacy and entered into the eMAR. Practically everything we do is a system.

A clinical information system is an arrangement of patients and the patient's medical team, data, processes, and information technology that interact to collect, process, store, and provide as output the information needed to care for a patient.

A clinical information system is not only data processing. A clinical system is also the interaction of people and technology to provide information that patient's medical team needs to do something.

Clinical information systems include:

- A transaction processing system that captures and processes information about a transaction such as entering and processing medical orders.
- MIS reports of the transaction such as the results of a patient's treatments.
- Decision support systems to help managers make decision such as when to increase or decrease staffing on a unit.
- An expert system provides expert advice such as IBM's Watson, which competed on *Jeopardy!*
- Communications and collaboration systems that enable people to share ideas such as email.
- Office automation systems such as Microsoft Office products that improve workflow.

Chapter 3 Clinical Database Analysis

A clinical database application is a computer program that is used to store and retrieve patient information or information necessary for patient care. Commonly used clinical database applications include an EMR, eMAR, CPOE, and an order management system.

A clinical database application consists of:

- A user interface: A user interface is a computer program that enables the clinician to store, retrieve, edit, and delete clinical information.
- A database management system (DBMS): A DBMS is a computer application that manages information stored in the database.
- Databases: A database is an electronic filing cabinet that contains clinical information.

The user interface is the portion of the clinical database application that you can see. The DBMS, the database, and information are stored in the database you cannot see because these are in a remote location connected to your computer by a computer network.

Clinical information is never deleted. Instead, the information is marked as a strike and amended, indicating that the information was corrected. The incorrect information remains but is not active.

A clinician enters a request for information into the user interface. The request is sent to the DBMS, where the request is processed, and information is returned and displayed on the computer screen by the user interface. For example, a nurse requests a list of patients who are on the nurse's unit by entering the unit's name into the user interface. The DBMS searches the database for patients on the specified unit and returns information about those patients to the user interface, where the information is displayed on the computer screen.

Chapter 4 Clinical Data Reporting

Clinical applications developed by third parties have built-in reports available from within the application. The clinician can select the built-in report and specify filtering criteria that remove all but selected information from the report. The report itself is designed by the clinical software vendor and cannot be modified by the clinician.

Some third-party vendors permit the healthcare facility's MIS department access to the clinical database enabling the clinical analyst to create custom reports using either a report writing tool such as Crystal Report or Structured Query Language (SQL) to retrieve clinical information from the database.

A report writing tool is a computer application that enables the clinical analyst to generate a report by using the report writing tool's user interface. The report writing tool then interacts with the clinical database to retrieve clinical information and format the clinical information into the report format designed by the clinical analyst.

In contrast, SQL is not a computer application. Rather, it is a type of programming language specifically designed to interact with DBMS to retrieve and manipulate information in the clinical database. SQL is the database language used by clinical software to interact with the clinical database. A clinical analyst who is familiar with SQL and has rights to interact with the DBMS can use SQL to generate reports and to manipulate the clinical database directly without having to use the clinical application.

Although many clinical software applications are licensed from third-party vendors and then tailored to the needs of the healthcare facility by the clinical analyst, a clinical analyst with a team of MIS developers may create a custom clinical database application. Chapter 2 discusses techniques needed to translate an idea for a clinical system into clinical specifications. Chapter 3 explores how to translate clinical specifications into a physical data model for the clinical database. This chapter discusses SQL statements that enable you to translate the physical data model into a working database. In addition, the chapter discusses how to store, retrieve, and manipulate information in the database.

Chapter 5 Clinical Project Management

A project is a temporary set of activities that delivers a unique outcome. A project is temporary, requires resources, is unique, and has a project sponsor who requested that the project be undertaken. Project management is applying project management skills and tools to transform an idea into reality. Project management skills and tools include a methodology to manage the transformation. The methodology is a set of proven techniques used to increase success and minimize risk during the transformation.

In this chapter, you will learn about tools used by project manager to apply a methodology that turns an idea into reality. These tools include:

- Project charter: A project charter specifies what the project manager is to deliver and the terms under which the project manager will manage the project.
- Scope statement: A scope statement is a brief expression of what will be delivered.
- The work plan: The work plan is a detailed description and organization of tasks and resource that are necessary to complete the project.
- Gantt chart: A Gantt chart is a visual depiction of the work plan.
- Critical path analysis: The critical path analysis determines tasks that will affect the duration of the project. That is, a change in duration of tasks that fall on the critical path affects the duration of the project.
- Cost estimates: A cost estimate is the project manager's projected cost of the project.

Chapter 6 Clinical Informatics Team Management

The project manager is the manager of the project and the project team. The project manager is also the facilitator of the project-coordinating project activities with the project sponsor, the stakeholders, and the project team to ensure that expectations are well defined and objectively measurable and that the project team delivers a system that meets the expectations of the project sponsor and stakeholders.

The project team consists of various numbers of professionals with different skill sets. Many team members have cross-functional expertise, enabling them to contribute in multiple ways to the project. The number of team members and their skillsets vary depending on the nature of the project. Some members are on the team for the length of the project, but others join and leave the team after they make their contributions to the project.

The project manager is the single leader of the team who makes decisions about the project with advice from members of the team, the stakeholders, and the project sponsor. The project manager uses open problem-solving techniques to address challenges that arise during the project. Open problem-solving techniques require that all problems be shared among team members, which encourages each person to help solve problems. The team has collective goals and is mutually accountable for meeting expectations.

Chapter 7 Clinical Computer Networks

Think for a moment. How is a progress note entered into a patient's electronic medical record transmitted to the electronic medical record application database and then made available to practitioners throughout the healthcare facility—and possibly outside the healthcare facility? The answer is that the progress note and other patient information are transmitted electronically over a computer network.

A network is both a physical and wireless connection among computers similar to how roadways connect houses and communities together. Each computer has a unique address similar to the street address of a house. Patient information is placed into an electronic envelope addressed to the destination computer, and the envelope is placed on the networks traveling to the destination computer.

This simple description of a computer network help to frame the complexity of networking that is presented in this chapter. It is important for the nurse informatics specialist to have a working understanding of how a computer network functions and how information is transmitted within seconds over the network.

Chapter 8 Clinical Vendor Negotiations

Many direct and indirect tasks are required to provide patient care. Direct tasks are tasks that can be directly associated with patient outcomes such as nursing care, medications, and accommodations in the patient's room. An indirect task is a task that is in support of a direct task such as hiring a nurse, acquiring medication, and procuring and maintaining the electronic medical records application.

A task, regardless if the task is a direct or indirect task, is performed by a resource. That resource can be an employee of the healthcare facility or a vendor, sometime referred to as a contractor. For example, a healthcare facility can use employees to build and maintain an electronic medical records application or purchase an electronic medical records application from a vendor and engage the vendor to maintain the application.

There is a clear distinction between an employee and a vendor. Tasks performed by an employee are controlled by the healthcare facility. Administrators determine what tasks need to be done, when to do the tasks, and how to perform the tasks. Every detail of the task is controlled by administrators.

In contrast, the healthcare facility has practically no influence on the details of tasks beyond an agreement with a vendor. Administrators engage a vendor to produce an outcome of tasks such as to implement electronic medical records systems. Administrators specify conditions within which the vendor produces the outcome such as the time frame, cost, and access to the healthcare facility and other constraints. However, the vendor controls every aspect of all tasks that are necessary to achieve the desired outcome. The vendor hires vendor employees, engages other vendors commonly called subcontractors, and determines work schedules and work rules.

The nurse informatics specialist will be in a position to engage vendors on behalf of the healthcare facility and manage vendors throughout the length of the agreement. The nurse informatics specialist will initiate and oversee the procurement process, select vendors, negotiate with vendors, and execute a contract with the vendor. Furthermore, the nurse informatics specialist will manage the vendor during the life of the contract.

Chapter 9 Clinical Disaster Recovery

A disaster is a catastrophic event that may cause significant damage and the possible loss of life. Catastrophic events include fire, floods, and powerful storms that place the ability to care for patients at risk. With conversion from paper to electronic medical records, a healthcare facility is exposed to being unable to access patient information and process medical orders during a power failure.

Let's say a wind storm causes a power disruption to the healthcare facility. The initial problem is administering medication. Some healthcare facilities use a computer on wheels (COW), which is a cart that contains a computer and medication for a group of patients. The computer is used to access the electronic medical records system (eMAR). Medication draws on the COW are typically locked. Entering a code into the COW opens the drawer. The COW is powered by a rechargeable battery that has a limited life of maybe 4 hours. Drawers usually can also be opened with a key.

Electrical power is needed to power computers at the nurse's desk, recharge the COW, power the local area network, power the network server, power the application server where the eMAR program resides, and power the database server where patient information is stored (see Chapter 7). If one of those devices lacks power, then the nurse is unable to access the eMAR that contains information needed to administer medication to patients.

A disaster can have significant impact on the healthcare facility other than loss of power. For example, staffing is a critical issue. Are staff members able to come to the hospital during a disaster? Roads may be closed, staff members may experience personal disasters at home, and staff members may simply prefer to stay home rather than risk injury while going to work. The administration may be able to hold over the current shift; however, at some point, the current staff needs a break. No staff can work more than 16 hours. As a result, the healthcare facility will lack staff to care for patients.

Another concern is supplies. Food, linens, medications, and other material needed to care for patients may not be refurnished because vendors are unable to deliver goods to the healthcare facility. The longer the impact of the disaster, the higher risk the healthcare facility is unable to care for patients.

A disaster can also include failure of heating, ventilation, and air conditioning or loss of key employees because of injury on or off the job or called up for military service. A staff strike of the healthcare facility or a vendor can place the healthcare facility in disaster mode.

Chapter 10 Clinical Systems Security

Clinical systems security is a critical factor in providing healthcare because practitioners and other clinicians make treatment decisions that prevent or reverse life-threatening illness. Initially, the patient presents with a medical problem. The practitioner asks questions and performs a physical assessment.

The practitioner then reviews the patient's medical records that include medication, test results, and other pertinent information that helps the practitioner decide the course of treatment. The practitioner trusts that the patient's medical records are intact and accurate and contains information about that patient.

No longer are medical records handwritten notes by the practitioner in the patient's file folder. Today medical records are electronic, enabling patient information to be available at anytime, anywhere depending on the availability of the electronic medical records system. Medical records are no longer kept on long shelves behind the reception desk in the practitioner's office or in oversized looseleaf binders in the chart room on the medical unit. Patients' records are stored in a database server (see Chapter 1) accessed by desktop and mobile computers over a computer network (see Chapter 7).

No longer can you feel and touch the patient's medical record. No longer is the patient's medical record in the exclusive custody of the practitioner. Today the patient's medical record is stored at some remote location in a server that is overseen by nonclinicians. In some cases, the remote location is not owned by the healthcare facility.

This may seem disconcerting; however, the practice of storing sensitive information electronically in a remote location is commonplace in many industries because security controls can be uniformly imposed that provide at times greater security than is provided to the patient's medical records in a practitioner's office because there is a record of who accessed the information.

Electronic medical records are convenient to store and access and provides the opportunity to use state-of-the-art electronic protection of patient's records; however, there is also an increased risk for unauthorized access, identity theft, computer viruses, and denial of service attacks. Protection is provided by proxy servers, fire walls, encryption, and other means to secure the network, computing devices, and patient information.

chapter 1

Nursing Informatics

LEARNING OBJECTIVES

1. Clinical informatics applications
2. Brief history of computers
3. Inside a computer
4. Inside an application
5. A clinical system
6. Clinical systems development

KEY TERMS

American Recovery and Reinvestment Act	Order management
	Patient profile
Bus	Patient Protection and Affordable Care Act
Central processing unit	
Change theory	Primary storage
Cognitive theory	Program
Computerized physician order entry	Proposal
Electronic health record	Request for proposal
Electronic medication administration record	Runtime library
	Secondary storage
Input devices	Server
Meaningful use	System
Motherboard	Systems theory
Multitasking	Transaction processing system
Operating systems	Web-based application

Nursing informatics is the area of nursing that combines nursing, information, and computer sciences to manage information required for use in nursing practice. The American Nurses Association (ANA) defines *nursing informatics* as a specialty that integrates nursing science, computer science, and information science to manage and communicate data, information, knowledge, and wisdom in nursing practice. The ANA recognized nursing informatics as a specialty in 1992.

The goal of nursing informatics is to support decision making of patients, practitioners, and nurses through the use of structured information and technology with the goal of reducing errors, improving communication, and promoting the use of evidence-based practice in all specialties of nursing.

A nurse specializing in nursing informatics may become involved in all aspects of developing and implementing a clinical information system; therefore, nurse informatics specialists need to be well versed in:

- Management of clinical information technology (Chapter 1): Management of clinical information technology is the application of computer technology and management information systems (MIS) to the clinical setting.
- Clinical systems analysis (Chapter 2): Clinical systems analysis is the process of analyzing the needs for a clinical system based on the workflow of the healthcare facility. A **system** is a way of doing something. A clinical system performs tasks of a clinical workflow.

- Clinical database analysis (Chapter 3): Clinical database analysis is the process of transforming the data requirements of a clinical information system into a database design that efficiently stores clinical information for use by a clinical information application.

- Clinical data reporting (Chapter 4): Clinical data reporting enables the nurse informatics specialist to interact with the clinical database directly to extract clinical information for reports.

- Clinical project management (Chapter 5): Clinical project management enables the nurse informatics specialist to design a detailed plan on how to transform an idea into a working clinical information system.

- Clinical informatics team management (Chapter 6): Clinical informatics team management enables the nurse informatics specialist to manage the project team, the clinical project sponsor, and stakeholders throughout the project.

- Clinical computer network (Chapter 7): The clinical computer network is the electronic highway over which clinical information travels among computers. An understanding of clinical computer networks enables the nurse informatics specialist to perform an end-to-end analysis of a clinical information system.

- Clinical vendor contracts and negotiations (Chapter 8): The nurse informatics specialist is likely to be the key person within the healthcare facility to interact with vendors that supply hardware and clinical applications to the healthcare facility. As a result, the nurse informatics specialist should have a firm understanding of contracts and negotiation strategies.

- Clinical disaster recovery and continuity (Chapter 9): A paperless clinical information system places increased dependency on electricity for the healthcare facility. Clinicians are unable to access the patient's electronic medical records, electronic medical administration records, and medical orders during a power failure. The nurse informatics specialist must be able to develop and enact a disaster recovery and continuity plan.

- Clinical systems security (Chapter 10): Regulatory requirements demand that patients' medical records be protected against unauthorized access. Electronic medical records that are accessible over the clinical computer network pose a risk. The nurse informatics specialist must understand how to protect patients' electronic medical records.

The Basis of Nursing Informatics

There are three theories that form the basis of nursing informatics. These are:

- **Systems theory**: Systems theory focuses on the interactions between the use of technology and systems of the human body.
- **Change theory**: Change theory focuses on implementing change from manual systems to technology-based systems within the healthcare environment.
- **Cognitive theory**: Cognitive theory focuses on the input, output, and processing necessary to accomplish the goal of a system.

At times there can be a confusion between the role of the management information system (MIS) and the role of nursing informatics because both focus on providing computerization of clinical workflows. MIS is responsible for applications, computer hardware, networking, security, and everything else involved in providing MIS to the entire healthcare facility.

Nursing informatics focuses on clinical applications primarily by analyzing clinical workflows, assessing the capabilities of clinical applications, and integrating clinical application into the healthcare facility's clinical workflow. In addition, the nursing clinical informatics specialist assists in developing policies and procedures related to clinical workflows and joins committees on **meaningful use** and core measurement, which are used by regulatory bodies to measure the performance of the healthcare facility.

Nursing informatics is frequently part of the MIS organization and is staffed by nurses who have had substantial clinical experience both as first-line healthcare provider and in administration. Furthermore, the nursing informatics specialist has the necessary MIS training in clinical systems analysis, clinical database analysis, and clinical project management. The combination of MIS and clinical skills places the nursing informatics specialist in a unique position to improve clinical workflows through computer automation.

Meaningful Use

The federal government is the key driver for implementing technology in healthcare facilities with the passage of the **Patient Protection and Affordable Care Act** and the **American Recovery and Reinvestment Act** of 2009 (ARRA).

The healthcare delivery system has lagged behind other industries in automating processes and realizing efficiencies for computerizing operations. Some researchers believe that resistance to technology is based on the cost of computerization and the challenge of changing multiple healthcare disciplines that work within an environment of autonomy. The lack of efficiencies that are prominent in other industries is seen as an area to recapture savings, especially by third-party payers such as the Centers for Medicare and Medicaid Services (CMS). However, healthcare providers need to automate their processes for CMS and other third-party payers to realize savings.

The ARRA provides financial incentives for hospitals and healthcare providers to convert paper systems to computerized systems. A total of $19 billion has been set aside to reimburse hospitals and healthcare providers for expenses related to automating clinical systems. The ARRA also provides a disincentive for maintaining paper-based systems. That is, reimbursement for Medicare patients to the hospital and healthcare provider will decrease if the hospital and healthcare provider do not automate their systems.

To receive reimbursement, hospitals and healthcare providers must show that the new technology is used in a meaningful manner. Specifically, hospitals must implement and use electronic health records (EHRs), computerized physician order entry (CPOE), order management, and electronic medication administration record (eMAR).

- **Electronic health record**: The EHR enables the staff to enter, store, and retrieve patients' medical records using a computer system.

- **Computerized physician order entry**: CPOE enables practitioners to enter orders directly into a computer. The CPOE system then transmits orders to the order management system for processing.

- **Order management**: The order management system enables staff to enter, store, and retrieve medical and nonmedical orders. In addition, the order management system interacts with other systems to receive and process orders.

- **Electronic medication administration record**: The eMAR system enables staff to enter, store, and retrieve medication orders and document medication administration. The eMAR system also interacts with the electronic pharmacy system to track inventory and billing for medication.

- **Patient profile**: A key element of the EHR is the patient profile. The patient file consists of a standard set of information that is maintained for every patient that can be exchanged with and updated by any healthcare provider who is caring for the patient.

NURSING ALERT

Meaningful use mandates seek to improve quality, safety, communication, and coordination of healthcare.

Responsibilities of Nursing Informatics

There is a fine line between MIS and nursing informatics. MIS is a division of the healthcare facility responsible for all computer software and hardware as well as data security and computer networks. Nursing informatics focuses on redesigning clinical workflows around technology, standardizing content across all healthcare informatics systems, analyzing the clinical needs of the healthcare facility, modifying vendor software to meet the changed workflows, being a catalyst for change within the healthcare facility, and encouraging evidence-based care throughout the facility using technology.

The nurse informatics specialist takes on the role of:

- Consultant: Advises both MIS and clinicians on how to use technology in the clinical environment.
- Analyst: Assesses the clinical need for technology and finds the best technology to meet those needs.
- Educator: Trains the clinical staff on the use of technology and the MIS staff on the clinician's needs.
- Policy developer: Incorporates technology in the facilities policies and procedures.
- Systems integrator: Ensures that all clinical systems are able to work together.
- Researcher: Identifies new technological solutions to clinical problems.

1. Clinical Informatics Applications

Clinical informatics application is a computer **program** that enables a person to enter, store, and retrieve clinical information, which is the fundamental function of many computer application that are used in other industries. The goal of an application is to automate a manual process. There are various manual processes to perform the same clinical task, and therefore there are many applications that automate the same task.

There are four options available to automate a manual process:

- Customized application: A customized application is an application that has been created to meet the specific needs of the healthcare facility. The customized application mimics the healthcare facility's manual process, requiring minimum training and change in the workflow.

- Off-the-shelf application: An off-the-shelf application is an application that is purchased from a vendor, and the application cannot be modified by the healthcare facility. The healthcare facility is likely required to adopt the workflow built into the vendor's application.

- Tailored application: A tailored application is an application that is purchased from a vendor and can be tailored to fit the workflow of the healthcare facility. The application is divided into two components, a core component and a modifiable component. The core component contains the processing logic of the application, and the modifiable component contains elements that can be changed by the healthcare facility, typically including nomenclature, screens, and limited processing such as required information. The healthcare facility will likely adjust some but not necessarily all workflows to accommodate the application.

- Open source: An open source application is an application that is built by an open source initiative in which volunteers develop a portion of the application. Anyone can download and use the application free of charge as long as they abide by the open software foundation license that, among other limitations states that you cannot charge for components of the open source application. The controversy surrounding open source applications is that some MIS professionals believe there is no one company that supports the application, although there are commercial companies that provide such support for a fee. Other MIS professionals believe greater support is available at no cost over the Internet because a community of developers built the application.

Few healthcare facilities choose the customized application primarily because of the expense and expertise required to create the application. Many healthcare facilities choose a tailored application or an off-the-shelf application depending on their needs and available financial resources. An off-the-shelf application is usually less costly and requires fewer support staff than the tailored application. However, the tailored application offers flexibility not available in the off-the-shelf application.

NURSING ALERT

Core components of a tailored application can be changed by the vendor; however, vendors usually require a committee of customers to agree to the change, which can be time consuming and frustrating to a healthcare facility that requests the change.

Application License

Applications are licensed and not sold to healthcare facilities. A license is a right to use the application under specific terms of the license. A license can be granted on a per computer basis using the application based on the full-time equivalent (FTE) clinical employees at the healthcare facility or by the number of concurrent users. Concurrent users means that number of employees who can use the application simultaneously.

Licenses are renewable after a period of time such as a year. The license renewal usually includes incremental upgrades to the application. However, an additional fee may be required for major upgrades to the application. A major upgrade may consist of features not available on the original version of the application.

The license usually carries a warranty. The warranty may state that the application meets current regulatory compliance and that compliance will be maintained throughout the licensing period. That is, the vendor is responsible for the application's meeting all government and regulatory specifications.

The vendor provides the healthcare facility with executable copies of the application and the database organized to facilitate storage of patient's records. Furthermore, the vendor may provide the healthcare facility with tools to modify the modifiable portion of the application. The core application cannot be modified by the healthcare provider. Any attempt to do so will void the warranty and license.

The database might be accessible to the healthcare facility. That is, a programmer might be able to generate customized reports directly from the database. However, the vendor frequently sets limitations on what the healthcare facility can do with the database. Violating the limitations may void the warranty and the license.

NURSING ALERT

The healthcare facility should have the MIS department and the legal department carefully review the license agreement before entering into a contract with a vendor.

Caution

Changing vendors after the healthcare facility implements a vendor's application is time consuming, costly, and challenging to accomplish. It is best to perform careful analysis of a vendor's product and licensing terms before contracting with a vendor.

2. Brief History of Computers

A computer is a device that can do two things. These are addition and subtraction. It is amazing how scientists and engineers are able to develop sophisticated electronics that can seem to do practically anything imaginable while still limited to basic addition and subtraction.

The first successful computer was developed in 3000 BC and was called the abacus. An abacus is a mechanical computer that uses rows of beads to represent numbers; moving a bead in one direction adds values and in the other direction subtracts values. It wasn't until the 17th century that Blaise Pascal, a French mathematician, developed a mechanical adding machine. The machine was called the Pascaline and used wheels and gears to perform addition and subtraction based on the same principle used in the abacus.

Charles Babbage expanded Pascal's concept and designed the difference engine and the analytical engine, which could multiply and divide as well as perform addition and subtraction. You'll remember from elementary school that multiplication and division are derived from addition and subtraction. The difference engine and the analytical engine were never built because they simply cost too much.

It wasn't until the turn of the 20th century that Herman Hollerith created the first electrical computer that used punch cards to read data and later instructions. His company was called the Tabulating Machine Company, which later changed its name to the International Business Machines Corporation (IBM).

In 1937, Dr. John Atanasoff and Clifford Berry, a professor and Atanasoff's graduate student, at Iowa State University created the first electronic computer that used vacuum tubes to store information and perform mathematical calculations. A vacuum tube is an electronic switch. The computer was called the ABC computer. They were also the first people to apply the binary numbers system to store and manipulate information (see Inside a Computer).

In 1946, Dr. John Mauchly of the University of Pennsylvania used the technology developed by Atanasoff and Berry to build the first generation of computers called the Electronic Numerical Integrator and Computer (ENIAC). The ENIAC had one purpose, which was to create accurate trajectory tables for the Department of Defense. Five years later, Mauchly built the Universal Automatic Computer, better known as the UNIVAC 1, for the Remington-Rand Corporation, which became the first well-known commercial electronic computer.

The second generation of computers ushered in when scientists at Bell Laboratories in New Jersey developed the transistor. The transistor provided the same electronic switching capabilities as a vacuum tube but at lower power, a reduced size, and lower cost. Computers were referred to as mainframe computers, took up floors of office buildings, and required a highly controlled environment to operate within.

The third generation of computers was launched in the mid-1960s with the discovery of integrated circuits. Hundreds of transistors that populated second-generation computer circuit boards were reduced to a circuit the size of a pin head. Computer manufacturers were then able to build smaller, more powerful, and less expensive computers and second-generation computers.

The year 1963 saw the first challenge to mainframe computers. Digital Equipment Corporation introduced the first minicomputer, called the PDP-8. A minicomputer was to some degree a scaled-down version of a mainframe computer in size, power, and price. For around $20,000 in 1963 dollars, a business could harness the power of a computer to run a portion of its operation.

Fourth-generation computers were born in 1971 with the introduction of large-scale integrated circuits. Large-scale integrated circuits technology enabled an entire computer circuitry to be placed on one computer chip. Four years into the fourth-generation computers, the first personal computer was introduced, called the Altair 8800. The Altair was designed for hobbyists. However, a few years later, more refined personal computers entered the market, including the Apple computer. It wasn't until 1981 that personal computers were taken seriously by the business community when IBM launched its own personal computer with the aid of Microsoft and Intel. IBM set the standard for personal computers.

The year 1984 was another turning point in the history of computers. It was the year when the first commercial graphical user interface was introduced for the Macintosh line of Apple computers. Microsoft followed the next year with the introduction of Windows. Computers became easier to use than previously because users clicked on icons rather than typing commands at a prompt.

In the 1960s, the Advanced Research Project Agency Network (ARPANET) was developed to connect together computers at remote research universities over an electronic network. This later evolved into the Internet. The Internet became available to others in the 1990 with the birth of the World Wide Web. Tim Berners-Lee developed the hypertext markup language (HTML), the uniform resource locator (URL), and the hypertext transfer protocol (HTTP). Collectively, these enabled information to be easily exchanged over the Internet. The following year Berners-Lee founded the W3 Consortium, which coordinates development of the World Wide Web. In 1993, the first commercial web browser called Mosaic was released, providing graphical access to the World Wide Web.

In 1973, Robert Metcalfe developed the first computer network called Ethernet. Ethernet enabled computers to be electronically connected and able to transfer information between computers.

3. Inside a Computer

Computers have the same general components regardless of size, power, and cost, and computers can add and subtract. In a sense, a computer is a box of switches. Information is stored by turning the switch on or off. At first this doesn't seem capable of storing more than two pieces of information, on or off. However, much more information can be stored in the computer by logically combining multiple switches together and using the binary numbering system to represent information.

The binary number system has two digits, 0 and 1. This is referred to as a base 2 numbering system. The term *base* refers to the number of digits in the numbering system. We normally use a base 10 number system. That is, the numbering system has 10 digits from 0 to 9. When we go beyond 9, we carry over 1 to the next place and start over such as 10. We recognize this as the number 10. Notice that the first column is a zero because we start with the first digit in the first position.

The same process of carrying over occurs with a base 2 or binary numbering system. The binary numbering system has two digits, 0 and 1. When we go beyond 1, we carry over to the next place and have 10. This may look like the number 10, but it is really the binary number 2. A binary digit is called a *bit*.

> **NURSING ALERT**
>
> The binary numbering system provides an understanding of how information is stored in a computer. You won't have to perform calculations using the binary numbering system.
> Any value that can be represented in our base 10 numbering system can be represented in the binary numbering system. Any calculation that can be performed using base 10 numbers can be performed using binary numbers.

Encoding Information

A switch has two states, off and on. Each state can represent a binary number. Off is 0, and on is 1. Several switches can be used to store a number, such as a nurse's salary, in a computer. Likewise, changing the setting of the switch can change the value of the number similar to moving the beads in an abacus.

Engineers organized switches into a set of eight switches called a byte. The largest number that can be represented in a byte is 255 decimal value or in binary 11111111. This still doesn't seem large enough; however, engineers combine bytes to represent larger values. Two bytes can hold 65,535 and four bytes 4,294,967,295.

Notice that all the numbers mentioned are whole numbers. None of them has fractional values. That's because fractional values are handled differently than whole numbers. Numbers that contain a fractional value are referred to as *floating-point numbers*. A floating-point number has two components. The first component consists of all the digits in the numbers, both the whole and fractional amounts. The second component is a number that implies the position of the separator.

The state of electronic switches is indicated by binary digits. A 0 implies an off state, and a 1 implies an on state.

You probably can see how numbers are stored inside a computer, but you're probably wondering how text is stored. Text is the more commonly stored information in a computer. Text includes numbers not used in calculations such as house numbers, punctuation marks, dollar signs, and other symbols on the keyboard.

Engineers devised a coding standard that translates letters, numbers, and symbols to a number value called the American Standard Code for Information Interchange (ASCII). One of up to 255 values is assigned to letters and symbols. Table 1–1 contains a sample of the ASCII code.

Each letter of the alphabet is represented twice in the ASCII code, once in upper case and again in lower case. To convert "Jim" into ASCII code, look up in the ASCII table the decimal number for an uppercase J, which is 74. Use the same procedure to locate the lowercase ASCII numbers for "im," which are 105 and 109, respectively. The equivalent decimal number can easily convert the decimal number to a binary number. The binary number can be easily stored in computer memory. Table 1–2 shows the conversation process.

A program reads the location in computer memory where the numeric equivalent of "Jim" is stored and interprets the numeric values as ASCII code. That is, the program translates the ASCII code into the letter, number, or symbol and then displays the name "Jim."

There is an inherent problem with the ASCII code. There aren't sufficient numbers available to accommodate symbols used in every language such as Asian languages that use ideographs. This problem was solved with the introduction of Unicode.

TABLE 1–1   A Sample of the ASCII Code

ASCII Value	Character	ASCII Value	Character	ASCII Value	Character
32	SPACE	64	@	96	'
33	!	65	A	97	a
34	"	66	B	98	b
35	#	67	C	99	c
36	$	68	D	100	d
37	%	69	E	101	e
38	&	70	F	102	f
39	'	71	G	103	g
40	(	72	H	104	h
41	)	73	I	105	i
42	*	74	J	106	j
43	+	75	K	107	k
44	,	76	L	108	l
45	-	77	M	109	m
46	.	78	N	110	n
47	/	79	O	111	o
48	0	80	P	112	p
49	1	81	Q	113	q
50	2	82	R	114	r
51	3	83	S	115	s
52	4	84	T	116	t
53	5	85	U	117	u
54	6	86	V	118	v
55	7	87	W	119	w
56	8	88	X	120	x
57	9	89	Y	121	y
58	:	90	Z	122	z
59	;	91	[	123	{
60	<	92	\	124		
61	=	93	]	125	}
62	>	94	^	126	~
63	?	95	_		

TABLE 1–2 Converting the Name Jim to the Equivalent Binary Value		
Letters	**ASCII Decimal Value**	**Equivalent Binary Value**
Jim	74 105 109	01001010 01101001 01101101

Unicode contains two distinct blocks of code. One is called Unicode-2 and the other is Unicode-4. Unicode-2 uses a 16-bit (2-bytes) number to represent symbols. This means 65,536 distinct symbols can be assigned a Unicode-2 value.

However, there might be an occasion when a language contains more than 65,536 symbols. In this case, Unicode-4 is used for the additional symbols. Unicode-4 uses a 32-bit (4 bytes) number, which can handle about 1 million symbols. The most commonly used symbols in every language are assigned a Unicode-2 number. Therefore, most of the textual information is stored using 2 bytes per symbol. Unicode-4 symbols are inserted where necessary into the information.

Although Unicode accommodates every language, it does have a major drawback when used to represent English. Unicode requires nearly double the storage space compared with the same English text represented by ASCII code.

Not all symbols used in Unicode or ASCII code are visible. Some symbols such as tab, linefeed, and carriage return are nonprintable symbols. This means you can include these symbols in the textual information, but you cannot see them on the screen or when the text is printed. Nonprintable symbols are commonly called *control characters*. For example, two characters are entered in the text whenever you press the Enter key. These are the linefeed and carriage return characters. A control character is a character embedded in a document that has a special meaning to a device such as ejecting a page from a printer. The linefeed character tells the video adapter or printer to move the cursor to the next line. The carriage-return character instructs the device to move the cursor to the beginning of the line. It is the responsibility of the device to recognize a control character and then translate the character into the appropriate action.

Instructions

The brain of a computer is the central processor. The central processor is a computer chip that has circuits designed to process information based on instructions. Each central processor type recognizes a set of instructions called an *instruction set*. The instruction set will have instructions to get a value (i.e., data) from a particular memory location, add the value, subtract the value, or store the value to a particular memory location. Today's central processors have a verbose set of instructions they can follow.

Processing Instructions

The mouse or the keyboard is used to indicate that you want to run a program. This sends an interrupt to the central processor. The central processor stops what it is doing and then looks up the interrupt type on the interrupt vector table. The interrupt vector table contains the memory address of the interrupt service routine. An interrupt service routine is a program the processor runs whenever an interrupt message is received. A common request is for the processor to run a program. The name of the program is either entered in the Run dialog box or is associated with an icon on the desktop.

After the program is selected, an interrupt is sent to the central processor to run the interrupt service routine that loads the requested program into memory. When in memory, the central processor receives the memory address of the first instruction of the program. The central processor examines the contents of the address and determines if the whole or partial instruction is received. If the instruction is incomplete, the central processor looks at the next address in sequence, which usually contains the other portion of the instruction. Next, the central processor determines if data is required to complete the instruction. If so, then the data is retrieved from the relative memory address before the central processor processes the instructions.

The results of the process is temporarily stored in memory called a *register* inside the central processor until the instruction is fully processed at which time the result is either stored in main memory or sent to the video display adapter where the result is displayed on the screen based on instruction from the program. When the last instruction is processed, the central processor waits for the next request to arrive.

The Motherboard

The **motherboard** is the largest circuit board inside the computer that contains many components, two of which are memory chips and the processor (Figure 1–1). Memory chips store instructions and data. These instructions tell the processor how to process the data. Each motherboard has characteristics that distinguish it from other motherboards. The most prominent of these are the form factor (which is the shape of the motherboard), the chipset, the bus, and the power supply.

A chipset consists of large-scale integrated circuits that make the motherboard come alive by coordinating the activities of the circuits and components that are integrated into the motherboard.

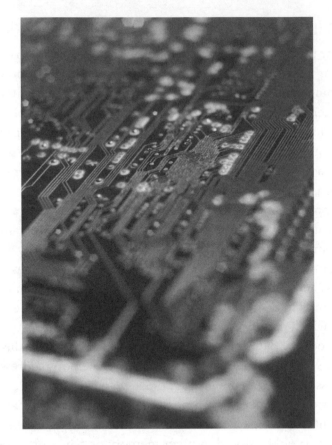

FIGURE 1–1 • The computer motherboard contains many components connected by etched wire.

A **bus** is the electronic pathway etched into the motherboard over which instructions and data flow to components. A bus is defined by two critical measurements. These are width (number of wires) and speed (the clock speed). Each wire on the bus carries 1 bit at a time; therefore, the more writes on the bus, the more bits can be available for the central processor to process at a time. Bits move over the bus in pulses generated by a clock. The higher the clock speed, the more pulses per second and the faster bits move over the bus. A bus is divided into two segments. One segment is used to transport addresses of components such as a memory address and the other transports data.

The Central Processor

Four important features define a central processor. These are processing speed, instruction set, memory cache, and the size of the information that can be read or sent at the same time.

The processing speed is the speed at which the central processor performs calculations and moves information inside the central processor. Speed is determined by a clock built into the central processor and functions similar to the clock on the motherboard except it affects only bits inside the central processor.

The instruction set is the group of commands that the processor understands. More powerful central processors have a robust instruction set and require fewer instructions from the program to process information. As a result, processing speed increases because the central processor has fewer needs to access memory.

Memory cache is memory inside the central processor that is used to temporarily store instructions, data, and results of calculations. Think of memory as a group of electronic switches that can be turned on or off (see Encoding Information). The more memory cache inside the central processor, the fewer times the central processor must temporarily store data outside the central processor.

The size of information that can be read or sent at the same time is referred to as a *word*. This is the number of bits that the central processor can receive in one pulse of the clock. The more bits that can be accepted by the central processor per pulse, the faster the information can be processed.

Display Memory

Information processed by the central processor is frequently displayed on the video display. Inside the computer, memory is reserved for the display sometimes called display memory. Whenever instructions call for information to be displayed on the screen, the central processor sends the information to the display memory.

Software called a display driver constantly reads display memory, transforming the binary values into picture elements called pixels that are displayed as an image on the screen. The resolution of the display is expressed as the width and height measured in pixels. For example, 1024 × 768 means the width is 1024 pixels and the height is 768 pixels. The higher the number of pixels, the higher the resolution can be displayed on the screen. The number of bits per pixels (bpp) determines the number of colors that can be used to display the image. Twenty-four bpp can produce 16.8 million colors, commonly referred to as true color.

Storage

Information is stored in either **primary storage** or **secondary storage**. Primary storage is in computer memory directly available for use by the central processor. Secondary storage is referred to as external storage (Figure 1–2). Information stored

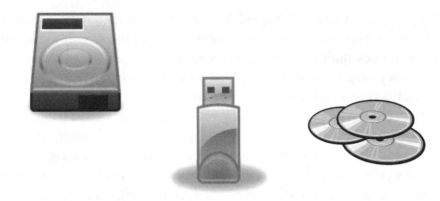

FIGURE 1–2 • Secondary storage includes disk drive, CD/DVD drives, and USB flash drives.

in secondary storage must first be loaded into primary storage for use by the central processor.

The most commonly used secondary storage device is the hard drive. The hard drive is an electromechanical device that encodes information on an electromagnetic medium using an arm moved by a motor. Information is stored in sections of the medium referred to as sectors. Information is retrieved by moving the arm to the appropriate sector and reading the value. Values are stored by adjusting the polarity of medium to represent 0 or 1.

USB flash drives are also common secondary storage devices. USB flash drives function similar to primary storage memory. CD and DVD disks use optical technology to store values 0 and 1 onto the medium. For large storage requirements, tape cartridges are used. A tape cartridge is stored in a tape library and is retrieved and inserted into a tape drive by a robotic arm.

The choice of secondary storage depends on the amount of information being stored and the speed at which the information needs to be retrieved. The fastest retrieval is memory. Therefore, applications that need almost instant access to information store information in primary storage.

> **NURSING ALERT**
>
> Many factors influence the speed at which information is retrieved, including network availability, database design, and the quality of instructions used to retrieve the information.

Input Devices

Various devices are used to input information into a computer. These devices are generally called **input devices** and include keyboards, mouse, and touch screens.

A keyboard is a set of switches that communicates your keystrokes in two ways. First, the keyboard tells the **operating system** which key or keys you selected. The keyboard also tells *you* that you successfully pressed the key. The keyboard is a small computer that runs a program to monitor all the keys and transmits a specific signal when one or several keys are pressed or released. Each key on the keyboard coincides with a position on a wired matrix inside the keyboard. Each matrix point has a unique key scan code. A portion of the operating system called the interrupt service routine interprets the key scan code into the equivalent ASCII value and then stores the ASCII value into main memory and erases the key scan code from the keyboard buffer.

A mouse is a pointing device consisting of the mouse and the mouse cursor, which appears on the screen. The mouse cursor appears in the default position on the screen when the computer turns on. The position is defined by coordinates on the screen. Moving the mouse tells the operating system to add or subtract to the existing coordinate and redraw the mouse cursor on the screen at the new coordinate.

Each time the mouse button is clicked and released, the operating system is notified of the action. The operating system sends all applications that are running the coordinates of the mouse cursor and whether or not the mouse button was clicked or released. In the case of Microsoft Windows, different messages are sent if the right or left mouse button was clicked or released. The application determines whether the coordinates correspond to its portion of the display and, if so, reacts appropriately to the action.

For example, if the coordinates correspond to the corner of the application's window and the right mouse button is clicked but not released, the application will resize the window according to the movement of the mouse.

A touch screen enables you to touch and move your finger on the screen to interact with elements on the screen. There are various technologies used by touch screens. These are:

- Capacitive touch screen: A capacitive touch screen holds the electronic charge at the point of contact. The operating system then reports the coordinates of that point to applications running on the computer. The application decides how to react.

- Resistive touch screen: A resistive touch screen increases resistance at the point of contact. The operating system then reports the coordinates of that point to applications running on the computer. The application decides how to react (Figure 1–3).

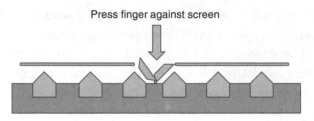

FIGURE 1–3 • Pressing your finger against the screen causes disruption in voltage, signaling the position on the screen.

- Infrared touch screen: An infrared touch screen divides the screen into a fine grid using beams of infrared light. Touching the screen causes the infrared beam to be broken at the point of contact. The operating system reports the coordinates of that point to applications running on the computer. The application decides how to react.

Operating System

An operating system organizes and controls hardware and software that resides on a computer (Figure 1–4). The most commonly used operating systems are Windows, the Macintosh operating system, and the UNIX operating system. There are two basic functions of an operating system. These are:

- Manage hardware and software sources in the computer.
- Provide a way for an application to deal with hardware by handing all the details for interacting with the central processor, memory, and other components inside the computer.

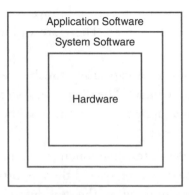

FIGURE 1–4 • The operating system manages applications and hardware inside the computer.

These functions are divided into six common tasks. These are:

- User interface: The user interface is the component of the operating system that you use to interact with the computer. Most user interfaces such as Windows and Mac OS are graphical user interfaces in which small images called icons are used to help the user navigate the computer. Nongraphical user interfaces are called command prompt user interfaces such as UNIX and require the user to type commands to navigate the computer.

- Application interface: The application interface is the component of the operating system that interacts with applications that run on the computer. This determines how the application is constructed to operate on the computer.

- Device management: The device management component is responsible for managing all devices connected to the computer such as monitors, mouse, keyboard, and network devices.

- Storage management: The storage management component is responsible for interacting with secondary storage devices to store information.

- Memory management: The memory management component is responsible for organizing and managing primary storage in the computer.

- Processor management: The processor management component is responsible for providing the central processor with instructions and data.

There are several types of operating systems. These are:

- Real-time operating system (RTOS): An RTOS is used to control machinery and has a skimpy user interface that enables the user to interact with the machine.

- Single-user, single-task operating system: A single-user, single-task operating system is designed to enable one person to do one thing at a time. The Palm operating system used for one of the original handheld computers called the Palm is an example of a single-user, single-task operating system.

- Single-user, multitasking operating system: A single-user, multitasking operating system is the most commonly used operating systems on personal computers. Operating systems such as Windows and Mac OS enable one person to do multiple things at the same time on the computer such as printing a document when writing another document in a word processor application.

- Multi-user operating system: A multi-user operating system enables many users access to the computer at the same time and is used on mainframe computers and shared computers called **servers**. UNIX, VMS, and MVS are examples of multi-user operating systems.

Multitasking

Multitasking implies that two or more tasks are performed by the computer at the same time such as printing a document while the user types into a word processor. To multitask, the central processor must be designed to perform multiple tasks simultaneously. Central processors used on personal computing devices can perform one task at a time; however, the operating system gives the feeling of multitasking by managing the central processor (Figure 1–5).

To understand how this works, it is important to understand what a task is. Consider typing text into a word processor. This seems like a task; however, a lot of subtasks are occurring and are managed by the operating system. For example, pressing a key on the keyboard is a subtask, as is releasing the same key. Although we usually don't recognize those as subtasks, the operating system does and treats each as an individual task.

A fraction of a second may transpire before keystrokes or maybe a few seconds depending how fast you type. During periods between keystrokes, no tasks are being sent to the computer. It is during these brief quiet periods that the operating system can send instructions from other applications to the central processor for processing. Processing happens so quickly that we get the feeling that more than one task is being performed by the computer at the same time. Some researchers refer to this as pseudo-multitasking because it appears that multitasking is happening, but the central processor is actually doing only one task at a time.

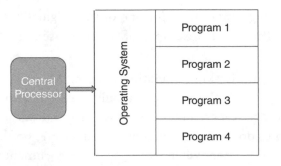

FIGURE 1–5 • The operating system gives the feeling of multitasking by sending instructions from each program to the central processor.

True multitasking occurs on multi-user computers such as servers that are shared among many users. A multi-user computer typically has multiple central processors to enable each to process different instructions. In addition, the systems administrator is able to give priority to certain users over other users. This is like letting the boss cut the line; however, the user is an application. For example, CPOE orders from the emergency department (ED), intensive care unit, and cardiac care unit will be processed before CPOE orders from a subacute unit.

Server

A server is a computer that is shared by multi-users over a computer network (see Chapter 7) (Figure 1–6). Typically, a server has robust capabilities that can meet high usage demands for a particular service. These services are:

- Database server: A database server is a computer that runs a database management system (DBMS) (see Chapter 3). Think of a database server as an electronic filing cabinet and the DBMS as the librarian who processes request for information and stores information in the library.

- Application server: An application server is a computer where applications are stored and distributed from when requested by users. For example, the eMAR application is stored on the application server rather than on each computer on the unit.

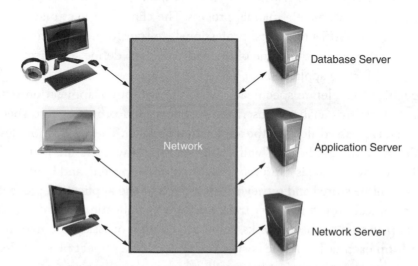

FIGURE 1–6 • Computers access the contents of a server by using the network.

- Mail server: The mail server is a computer that stores emails and contains an application that runs the email service for the organization.

- Print server: The print server is a computer that manage printing documents on printers that are located on the network. When print is selected by a user, the document is sent to the print server. Software on the print server sends the document to the designated printer.

- Network server: The network server is a computer that manages the computer network. It grants permission to use the network and routes network traffic to the desired destination.

- Web server: The web server is a computer that manages the organization's intranet (within the organization) and Internet (outside the organization).

- File server: The file server is a computer that enables multiple users to save and use files to the same disk. This is similar to a shared hard disk.

4. Inside an Application

The terms *software* and *program* are both used to describe a sequence of instructions that can be interpreted and executed by the central processor of a computer. In contrast, an application consists of one or more programs that collectively achieve a single purpose. For example, eMAR is an application that consists of multiple programs that collectively are used to document medication administration.

The application is born when the project sponsor initiates the project (see Chapter 5) to automate a manual process. The clinical project manager organizes a team of MIS and clinical professionals to transform the manual process to a computer application. One of the first tasks is to define specifications (see Chapter 2) for the application.

Specifications define specifically what the computer application is to do. A clinical systems analyst transcribes workflows and processes into specifications that are passed along to the application designer. The application designer decides how the application will work—that is, how users interact with the application; what data is captured, processed, and reported; and how the information will be stored and retrieved. All aspects of the application are laid out.

The clinical project manager transforms the specifications and design into a project plan that consists of tasks, subtasks, duration of tasks, resources needed to perform each task, and the cost of the project. The project plan is a detailed roadmap on how the project team will deliver the application.

Programmers and Programs

A programmer is a member of the project team who is responsible for translating specifications and design requirements into a program. The program contains explicit instructions to the **central processing unit** on what to do and when to do it. Think of this as writing steps in a recipe.

The programmer uses a high-level computer language to write the program. Many different programming languages are available. The programming language selected for the application depends on many technical factors. The language is referred to as a high-level computer language because the language is relatively easy for the programmer to learn and write. The central processor, however, only understands a low-level computer language that is challenging for the programmer to learn and write.

Instructions are written into an editor. An editor is a barebones word processor without any formatting capabilities. When you use a word processor, the word processor inserts many formatting characters into the document that you don't see, such as font style, size, and page markers. These characters are in the document. The program requires only instructions. Because these formatting characters will cause errors, the programmer uses an editor that only places what the programmer types into the file.

When the programmer has finished writing the program, the program is saved to a file called the source code file. *Source code* is a term used for the instructions written by the programmer. Source code cannot be read by the central processor because source code is written in a high-level language, and the central processor only understands low-level machine language.

A program called a *compiler* translates source code into the computer's native machine language. The compiler stops running if there is something in the source code that the compiler doesn't understand. This is referred to as a syntax error and is usually caused by a misspelling or a typographic error made by the programmer. The programmer then fixes the problem in the source code and recompiles the program.

Frequently, parts of the source code that are used in many programs are already compiled and saved to a library. The programmer references these parts by inserting an "include" statement into the source code. The "include statement" tells the compiler that the part needs to be included from the library. A program called a linker reads the include statement, retrieves the corresponding compiled part from the library, and links the part to the compiled program.

The compiler or linker produces an executable program that is readable by the central processor (Figure 1–7). The executable program is the program that

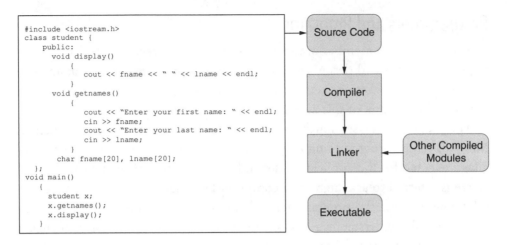

FIGURE 1–7 • Source code written by the programmer is then complied and linked into machine-readable code called the executable program.

is loaded onto the computer and loaded into memory when a user wants to run the application.

Testing

After the executable program has been installed on the computer, the programmer tests the program to determine if the program meets the specification. That is, does the program do what the programmer intends it to do? If so, then the programmer moves on to write the next program in the application.

Frequently, the program doesn't work correctly the first time because of a logic error. A logic error occurs when the process isn't working as expected even if the instructions are written correctly. This is like leaving out a step in the recipe. The recipe is written correctly, but one or more steps should have been included in the recipe.

This is commonly referred to as a bug in the program and is the cause of an application not working properly. As the lines of source code increase and more programs are added to the application, there is a greater risk that logic errors will arise. Testing the application before release of the application is expected to identify logic errors; however, some logic errors only materialize when the application is used in real life.

When a logic error is detected, the programmer must find the error, revise the source code, and compile and test the source code before releasing the revision to users. A revision is an update to the application that is released after the application is being used. Some releases fix bugs, and other releases provide enhanced features to the application.

Runtime Libraries

Components of some applications—in particular, Windows applications—are released as a **runtime library** rather than in an executable program. A runtime library has parts of the program that are not part of the executable program. When the executable program requires the component, the component is copied from the runtime library and linked into the executable program. Runtime libraries enable programmers to change and distribute a portion of the application without having to compile the complete application and distribute a large executable program.

On occasion, you might have seen an error message stating that the runtime library was not found. This means that the operating system could not locate the runtime library and cannot fulfill the request of the executable program. Sometimes the runtime library is not installed on the computer or the operating system doesn't know where to find the runtime library on the computer.

Web-Based Applications

A **web-based application** is an application that uses a variety of technologies to perform the application's objective. The application interface is a web page that is displayed by a browser on the user's computer. The web page contains text, images, and instructions on how they are to be displayed. In addition, some web pages have instructions on how to logically process information. The browser, which is an executable program, knows how to interpret the instructions and present the page on the screen. The programmer who writes the web page can have hyperlinks built into the web page enabling the user to display other web pages based on the workflow of the application.

The web page resides on a web server and is accessed by entering the address of the web server into the address bar of the browser or by using a hyperlink that contains the web server access. The initial request causes the web server to send the browser the index.html file, which is commonly referred to as the home page. From there, the browser can request specific pages at the request of the user of the application.

A web page can collect information from a user in the form of a web form. A web form is an electronic form displayed by the browser that collects information from the user and then submits the data to a common gateway interface (CGI) program that resides on the web server. The CGI program reads the incoming information and then processes the information based on instructions written by the programmer who wrote the CGI program. Many times the CGI program calls other applications such as a database application to process the information.

When processing is completed, the CGI program dynamically creates a web page containing the processed information and sends the web page to the browser, which displays the information on the screen. This is how a web page displays personal information about a user.

5. A Clinical System

A system is a way of doing something to achieve a desired result. A system can be a manual process such as driving to work, an electronic process such as documenting an admissions assessment in an electronic medical record, or a combination such as measuring blood glucose from a finger stick. Each of these is a system.

A system has four elements (Figure 1–8). These are:

- Input: Input is the activity of gathering data such as a blood sample.
- Processing: Processing is the activity of transforming data into a useful output such as the glucose meter measuring the blood sample.
- Output: Output is the production of useful information such as the blood glucose level in the sample of blood.
- Feedback: Feedback is adjustment, if any, to the input based on the output such as taking another blood sample if the blood glucose level is unusual.

An electronic clinical system is a system, primarily a computer-based system, in which data is entered into the computer using a keyboard, mouse, scanning device, or touch screen and processed by a program running on the computer. Output can be displayed on the screen, sent to a printer, stored in a

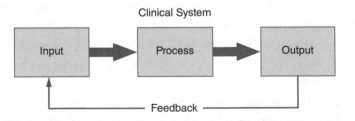

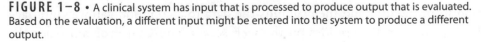

FIGURE 1–8 • A clinical system has input that is processed to produce output that is evaluated. Based on the evaluation, a different input might be entered into the system to produce a different output.

database, or transmitted through the computer network to another computer. Based on the output, different data might be reentered into the computer for processing.

Types of Systems

Nursing informatics focuses on electronic systems converting a manual system to a computerized system. Different types of systems are used in the healthcare industry. These can be generalized into the following types of electronic systems:

- Office automation system: An office automation system is designed to improve common activities in the office and includes word processing (i.e., Word), spreadsheet (Excel), email (i.e., Outlook), and other programs typically purchased from a vendor.

- Database system: A database system is a system that stores and retrieves data and is usually integrated with other types of systems.

- Transaction processing system: A **transaction processing system** captures, processes, and stores information. A patient admissions system is a transaction processing system because the system is used to collect, process, and store patient information.

- MIS: An MIS is designed to provide information to help the manager make decisions. For example, an MIS provides clinical managers with aggregate patient information needed to manage a clinical unit of the facility.

- Decision support system: A decision support system helps the manager make decisions by analyzing information stored in a database. For example, the ED's patient tracking system can alert the clinical manager and ED staff when a patient has been in the ED for 20 minutes and has yet to be assessed by a practitioner.

- Expert system: An expert system is designed to provide advice that would otherwise be offered by an expert. For example, a CPOE may recommend a set of admitting orders or display an alert if an order appears contrary to protocol.

- Artificial intelligence system: An artificial intelligence system has the ability to learn and to make decisions based on what the system has learned.

- Integrated system: An integrated system is a network of systems that interact with each other to provide nearly seamless processing. For example, an eMAR system, electronic medical record system, CPOE system, and electronic order management system are usually integrated so that input and processing can be shared appropriately among these systems.

- Inter-company systems: An inter-company system is able to share data between two independent organizations. For example, reimbursement information might be electronically shared by the healthcare facility with third-party payers using an inter-company system.
- E-commerce system: An e-commerce system is used to conduct business over the Internet.

Systems can be classified in the following ways:

- Open system: An open system requires human input. Most nursing informatics systems are open systems.
- Closed system: A closed system uses sensors as input and does not require humans.
- Adaptive system: An adaptive system can change based on the input.
- Nonadaptive system: A nonadaptive system is unable to change based on input.

The performance of a system is measured by performance standards.

Transaction Processing Systems

A transaction is an activity that has a beginning, processing, and an end. For example, a practitioner enters an order. The order is processed and sent to the destination department for processing. The practitioner then receives notice that the order is waiting to be executed. Collectively, these steps are a transaction.

Some transactions require multiple processing steps. The transaction is not completed until all steps in the process are completed successfully. For example, the CPOE order for medication must be sent to the unit, to the pharmacy, and to the billing department. If any of these steps fails, the order has failed to process. The practitioner then receives notice that the order has failed. Many nurse informatics systems are transaction processing systems, some requiring subsequent processing information by other applications.

Processing Methods

Processing is a series of steps that transforms information into another form such as transforming elements of a CPOE order into a form that can be stored into a database. Some processing requires calculations and other processing requires comparing information with information that exists elsewhere (i.e., login).

A processing method is the way processing occurs. There are two general kinds of processing:

- Batch processing: Batch processing is when all information that needs processing is stored, called batching, and the batch is processed at the same time. For example, a payroll is processed using batched processing because this is the most efficient way to process the information.

- Real-time processing: Real-time processing, sometimes referred to as transactional processing, is when information is processed as the information is received. Therefore, the processing result is immediate.

6. Clinical Systems Development

After a decision has been made to acquire a new clinical system, the MIS department prepares a **request for proposal** (RFP). An RFP is a formal document distributed to vendors asking each vendor to submit a **proposal** for delivering the new clinical system. The RFP must at least state:

- The problem: The RFP states the clinical problem that the proposed clinical systems will resolve.

- Expectations: Expectations specify how the MIS department perceives the new clinical system will work to resolve the clinical problem.

- Constraints: A constraint is a limitation within which the new clinical system will work such as having to work with the healthcare facility's current network capabilities.

- Timeline: The timeline specifies when the new clinical system needs to be up and running.

> **NURSING ALERT**
>
> Before distributing an RFP, the MIS department may distribute a request for information (RFI) to vendors. The RFI seeks general information about products and services offered by the vendor.

The Proposal

Each vendor that wants to provide the new clinical system must submit a proposal in writing to the MIS department. The proposal should include:

- Restate the clinical problem. This reassures that the vendor understands the problem that is to be remedied.

- Restate the MIS expectations. This too reassures that the vendor understands what MIS is expecting to receive when the new clinical system is delivered.

- MIS constraints reaffirm limitations imposed by the MIS department.
- Restatement of the MIS timeline.
- A description that the vendor understands how the current clinical system works.
- A description of how the vendor expects the new clinical system will function.
- Statement of realistic constraint identified by the vendor, such as cost, technology, and scheduling. For example, the vendor may require an upgrade of the facility's network.
- The vendor's timeline for delivering the new clinical system.
- Cost breakdown: Hardware and infrastructure cost, development cost, and ongoing maintenance cost.
- Ongoing staffing requirements by the healthcare facility.

Assessing Proposals and Products

Proposals can span a gamut of offers. Some are reasonable offers, while others might be extreme or incomplete. The steering committee, which is composed of the MIS department along with attorneys, accountants, and clinicians, evaluates each proposal and then either modifies the original RFP or negotiates terms with the vendors (see Chapter 8).

A proposal is likely from vendors that provide tailored products or off-the-shelf products. Tailored products enable the healthcare facility to modify a small portion of the application to conform to the healthcare facility's workflow. Off-the-shelf products cannot be modified, and the healthcare facility will have to modify its workflow to correspond to the workflow of the off-the-shelf product.

Evaluation of products should focus on:

- Functionality: Does the product address the clinical problem that the healthcare facility is trying to solve?
- Ease of use: Is the product easy to use?
- Reliability: Does the product provide consistent performance?
- Efficient use of resources: Does the product demand too much of the infrastructure and staff?
- Maintainability: Is the product easy to maintain by the vendor and MIS staff?
- Scalability: Can the product handle increases and decreases in volume without having to reprogram the application?

To answer these questions, the evaluation team can use a scenario approach to assess the product. The scenario approach is driven by a series of "what if" questions that pose likely and unlikely scenarios to evaluate how the product will work under those situations. The goal is to compare the product with a critical success factor. A critical success factor is an element that determines if the product will likely succeed. The goal is to find a showstopper—a missing critical success factor.

The steering committee must also consider the viability of the vendor. The vendor must be sustainable as a business because the healthcare facility's capability to deliver quality patient care greatly depends on the vendor's product, and the sustainability of the product depends on the vendor's capability to remain in business and provide the level of support required by the healthcare facility.

CASE STUDY

CASE 1

The executive nurse asks you to brief her on options for implementing an electronic medical record application for the healthcare facility. This is the first clinical application that the healthcare facility will adopt as part of the meaningful use incentives. The executive nurse is familiar with computer applications but is unfamiliar with acquiring and implementing an electronic medical record application. She asks you the following questions. What are your best responses?

QUESTION 1. Should the healthcare facility purchase an off-the-shelf application or acquire one that can be tailored to the healthcare facility's workflow?
ANSWER: Both options are feasible and will provide the healthcare facility with an electronic medical record application. The off-the-shelf application is limited because the healthcare facility is unable to modify the application. The healthcare facility will have to adopt the workflow used in the off-the-shelf application. In contrast, the tailored capable application enables the healthcare facility to possibly merge the healthcare facility's workflows with that of the application. However, the tailored capable application requires increased MIS staff to administer and modify the application.

QUESTION 2. How do we go about acquiring the application?

ANSWER: The initial step is to gather the general needs of the healthcare facility for an electronic medical record application and identify vendors that provide electronic medical record applications. Next, each vendor should be sent a request for information that contains those questions. After the information has been provided, the healthcare facility needs to write the specifications the healthcare facility requires of an electronic medical record and include the specifications in a request for proposal that is sent to vendors. Vendors that are interested in providing the application will submit proposals that will be reviewed by the healthcare facility.

QUESTION 3. Should the healthcare facility consider an open source electronic medical record application?

ANSWER: An open source application is built by an open source initiative and can be downloaded and installed at no cost to the healthcare facility. However, the MIS department will be responsible for the installation and operation of the application. Healthcare facilities that use open source applications typically engage a vendor that is familiar with the installation, configuration, and implementation of the open source application.

QUESTION 4. Should the healthcare facility purchase or license the electronic medical record application?

ANSWER: Nearly all applications are licensed by vendors and are not sold to healthcare facilities. A license grants the healthcare facility rights to use the application under the licensing terms. The license may be based on FTE clinical staff, number of concurrent users, or a charge per computer that uses the application. The license might be renewable each year.

FINAL CHECK-UP

1. **During a training session, a nurse asks you what meaningful use is. What is the best response?**
   A. Healthcare facilities are providers that receive reimbursement for electronic medical records if they show that they use the technology to improve patient care.
   B. Meaningful use is part of the Patient Protection and Affordable Care Act.
   C. Meaningful use is using electronic medical records to improve patient care.
   D. Healthcare facilities are provided with additional software if they use the electronic medical records to improve patient care.

2. **What is the role of a nurse informatics specialist?**

   A. A consultant, analyst, and nurse coordinator
   B. An educator, consultant, analyst, and researcher
   C. A policy developer, analyst, nurse supervisor, and programmer
   D. A programmer, analyst, MIS coordinator, and nurse

3. **A student nurse asks you what a systems integrator is. What is your best response?**

   A. Incorporates technology in the facilities policies and procedures
   B. Ensures that all clinical systems are able to work together
   C. Assesses the clinical need for technology and finds the best technology to meet those needs
   D. Identifies new technological solutions to clinical problems

4. **What is a system?**

   A. A system is a way of doing something to achieve a desired result.
   B. A system is a way of using a computer to do something to achieve a desired result.
   C. Computer hardware.
   D. Computer hardware and software.

5. **What is a transaction processing system?**

   A. A transaction processing system is designed to provide information to assist managers to make decisions.
   B. A transaction processing system captures, processes, and stores information.
   C. A transaction processing system stores and retrieves data and is usually integrated with other types of systems.
   D. A transaction processing system helps managers to make decisions by analyzing information stored in a database.

6. **What is an RFI?**

   A. A proposal
   B. Request for proposal
   C. Request for instruction
   D. Request for information

7. **What is scalability?**

   A. Recognizing that there is no one-size-fits-all application
   B. Choosing the most appropriate staff for the project
   C. Balancing the application's benefits and deficits
   D. The ability to increase and decrease in volume without having to reprogram the application

8. **What is real-time processing?**
   A. When information is processed as the information is received. The processing result is immediate.
   B. All processing is processed at the same time, and the result is immediate.
   C. All processing is processed at the same time, and the result is delayed.
   D. When information is processed as the information is received. The processing result is delayed.

9. **What is an application server?**
   A. A computer that manages the computer network
   B. A computer that runs a database management system (DBMS)
   C. A computer where applications are stored and distributed from when requested by users
   D. A computer that enables multiple users to save and use files to the same disk

10. **What is multitasking?**
    A. Two or more tasks are performed by the computer at the same time.
    B. Two or more tasks seem to be performed by the computer at the same time.
    C. A computer with two central processors.
    D. A computer with a single central processor.

CORRECT ANSWERS AND RATIONALES

1. A. Healthcare facilities are providers that receive reimbursement for electronic medical records if they show that they use the technology to improve patient care.
2. B. An educator, consultant, analyst, and researcher.
3. B. Ensures that all clinical systems are able to work together.
4. A. A system is a way of doing something to achieve a desired result.
5. B. A transaction processing system captures, processes, and stores information
6. D. Request for information.
7. D. The ability to increase and decrease in volume without having to reprogram the application.
8. A. When information is processed as the information is received. The processing result is immediate.
9. C. A computer where applications are stored and distributed from when requested by users.
10. A. Two or more tasks are performed by the computer at the same time.

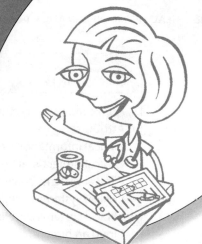

chapter 2

Clinical Systems Analysis

LEARNING OBJECTIVES

1. A clinical system
2. Clinical systems development process
3. Entities
4. Object-oriented design
5. Data capture
6. Application architecture

KEY TERMS

Application architecture	Object
Attributes	Primary key
Clinical information system	Project charter
Clinical project manager	Pseudo code
Clinical systems analyst	Scalability
Clinical systems designer	Scope statement
Clinical systems developer	Stakeholder
Cloud architecture	System
Data flow diagram	System owner
Entity	System user
Entity relationships	Thin client
Leveling diagram	Tiers
Method	Work breakdown structure

1. A Clinical System

A **system** is a group of interrelated components that function together to achieve a desired result. Simply said, a system is a way of doing something. It can be a manual process such as taking a telephone order from a practitioner. It can be an electronic process such as a computerized physician order entry (CPOE). Or it can be a combination of manual and electronic processes such as taking a telephone order that is processed by the pharmacy and entered into the electronic medication administration record (eMAR). Practically everything we do is a system.

A **clinical information system** is an arrangement of patients and the patient's medical team, data, processes, and information technology that interact to collect, process, store, and provide as output the information needed to care for a patient.

A clinical information system is not only data processing. A clinical system is also the interaction of people and technology to provide information that patient's medical team needs to do something.

Clinical information system includes:

- A transaction processing system captures and processes information about a transaction such as entering and processing medical orders.

- Management information system (MIS) that reports the transaction such as the results of a patient's treatments.

- Decision support systems that help managers make decision such as when to increase or decrease staffing on a unit.
- An expert system that provides expert advice such as IBM's Watson, who competed on *Jeopardy!*
- Communications and collaboration systems such as email, which enables people to share ideas.
- Office automation systems such as Microsoft Office products that improve workflow.

The Players

Each system has stakeholders. A **stakeholder** is any person who has an interest in an existing or proposed clinical information system. Every system has a **system owner**. A system owner is the sponsor or executive advocating for the system, the person who provides funding and controls the finished system. Systems have users. A **system user**, commonly referred to as the customer, uses the system or is affected by information generated by the system.

Each system has a team of developers. A developer is a person who makes the system a reality by identifying the clinical requirements and then building and implementing the clinical system that fulfills the clinical requirements.

The development team consists of:

- A **clinical project manager:** A clinical project manager is responsible for planning, building, and delivery of the completed project. The clinical project manager is also responsible for managing the project team.
- A **clinical systems analyst:** A clinical systems analyst is responsible for identifying the clinical requirements of the clinical system and translating clinical requirements into clinical specifications for the system.
- A **clinical systems designer:** A clinical systems designer is responsible for translating clinical specifications into technical specifications.
- A **clinical systems developer:** A clinical systems developer is responsible for building the clinical system based on technical specifications. A clinical systems developer may focus on a particular aspect of development such as databases, user interfaces, or back-end processing.

NURSING ALERT

It is common that one person will fill multiple roles in the development team.

The Clinical Systems Analyst

The clinical systems analyst is a problem solver and must:

- Identify problems—real or anticipated—that require corrective action in a clinical process.
- Identify opportunities to improve the process.
- Follow directives to change the process based on complaints.

A clinical systems analyst—the person who analyzes the clinical system—can be found in various areas of the organization, but typically a clinical systems analyst works in the management information systems (MIS) department.

The clinical systems analyst is the facilitator for everyone in the project and pulls together all information about the process from all stakeholders. The clinical systems analyst is the only person who knows the details of a process from beginning to end.

A clinical systems analyst takes a request for a system and transforms the request into reality by writing clinical specifications that inform the development team how the clinical system should operate. The clinical systems analyst's objective is to create clinical specifications for a clinical system that includes:

- Input screen design
- Details of clinical processes
- Storage and retrieval of clinical information

Furthermore, the clinical systems analyst must design the system to work within the system architecture. Think of the system architecture as the computer environment—computer, servers, and network.

The clinical systems analyst takes an idea and transforms the idea into reality.

2. Clinical Systems Development Process

The clinical systems development process begins with a request from the administration, usually to address change in procedure or a regulatory requirement or to take advantage of a new clinical opportunity. The clinical systems development process is a set of activities that develops and maintains clinical information systems and related software.

The process begins by using a problem-solving approach:

- The need is identified usually by administration.
- The need is studied by the systems analyst.

- Alternative solutions are identified and explored.
- The best solution—usually a modification to the clinical system or a new clinical system—is adopted.
- The clinical system is then designed, developed, and implemented.
- If the problem is not resolved with the implementation of the clinical system, then the problem-solving process begins again.

NURSING ALERT

Many clinical systems are designed and developed by third parties. A clinical systems analyst can use tools supplied by the vendor to modify the clinical system before the clinical system is implemented.

Expectations

It is important that the system owner, the stakeholders, and the development team have the same expectations. Two ways to ensure expectations are clear are to create a scope statement and a project charter.

The **scope statement** describes the common understanding of all deliverables such as the online order entry system that enables practitioners to enter medication orders from any computer.

The **project charter** is a contract between the system owner and the development team that defines expectations. The charter also specifies constraints within which the system is developed and operates. These might be technology limitations or financial limitations. The project charter is signed by the system owner and the project manager before work begins on the system.

The clinical systems development process begins in earnest after the project charter and scope statement are in place. The clinical systems development process is:

- System initiation: System initiation is the initial planning for the project that defines the project team, tasks, schedule, and budget.
- System analysis: System analysis is when clinical requirements are defined.
- System design: System design translates clinical requirements into technical specification.
- System implementation: System implementation is when the clinical system is built, tested, and installed.

Work Breakdown Structure

The challenge is how do you understand a clinical process in detail so that you can automate the process? The request for the clinical system is usually stated in a few words such as a yellow sticky note asking to build an online course registration system. Begin to learn about the process using the **work breakdown structure**.

The work breakdown structure is a process of decomposing a simple request into smaller components that are easy to comprehend and analyze.

Let's say you are asked to build a patient's electronic medical record. Begin with the whole—look at the outcome, the whole electronic medical record. Dissect the whole into logical components and then dissect each component into smaller components. These are called levels.

Levels are related using a number system; 1 is always the whole, and 1.1, 1.2, and so on are second-level components. The progression continues until we have a component that we can easily analyze. This is called a work package. The task is to define each work package and then create a system equivalent to the work package. All work packages are then assembled into the whole system. Figure 2–1 shows an example of a portion of the work breakdown structure for the electronic medical record.

Data Flow Diagram

A **data flow diagram**, also known as a context diagram, is used to analyze a work package. A data flow diagram is an illustration of a workflow (Figure 2–2). Symbols are used to define elements of the workflow. Here are symbols commonly used in a data flow diagram.

- A circle is a process.
- An arrow is a data flow.
- A rectangle is an element external to the system.
- Parallel lines are used to indicate a place to store data called a data store.

Leveling Diagram

A **leveling diagram** is another tool used to analyze a clinical process (Figure 2–3). A leveling diagram is a form of a data flow diagram at a level of detail in the process. Leveling diagrams are used to discuss the clinical process with stakeholders, each of whom may have a different view of the process.

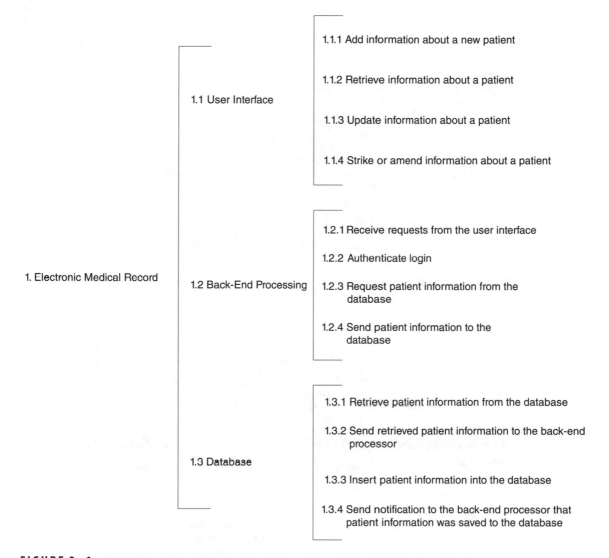

1. Electronic Medical Record

1.1 User Interface

1.1.1 Add information about a new patient

1.1.2 Retrieve information about a patient

1.1.3 Update information about a patient

1.1.4 Strike or amend information about a patient

1.2 Back-End Processing

1.2.1 Receive requests from the user interface

1.2.2 Authenticate login

1.2.3 Request patient information from the database

1.2.4 Send patient information to the database

1.3 Database

1.3.1 Retrieve patient information from the database

1.3.2 Send retrieved patient information to the back-end processor

1.3.3 Insert patient information into the database

1.3.4 Send notification to the back-end processor that patient information was saved to the database

FIGURE 2–1 • A simple work breakdown structure for an electronic medical record application.

For example, the director of nursing may be able to discuss the process at level 1. And the unit manager may be able to discuss the process at a lower level, which is more detailed than the previous level.

Use the commonsense rule when working with leveling diagrams. Stop at the level that makes sense for your system. The goal is for you to understand and be able to explain the clinical process, not to create levels upon levels of diagrams.

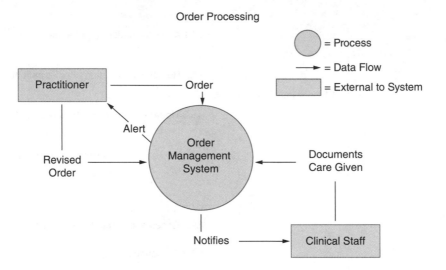

FIGURE 2–2 • A data flow diagram showing the workflow for entering and processing an order.

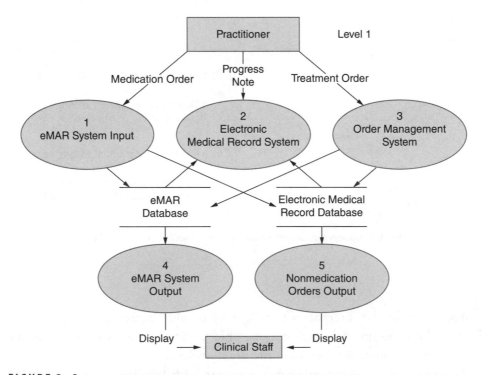

FIGURE 2–3 • A leveling diagram describing further details of the ordering process. eMAR, electronic medication administration record.

Pseudo Code

The goal is to define details of each clinical process using **pseudo code**. Pseudo code is a step-by-step description of the logical flow of a process. The clinical systems analyst can walk stakeholders step by step through the process, enabling stakeholders to correct anything that is unclear. The result is a major decrease in logical errors—bugs—in the system.

Pseudo code contains steps. Steps can be:

Sequential:
    Prompt the user to enter a user ID
    Prompt the user to enter a password
    Validate the password
IF-ELSE statements:
    If the medication is due within an hour then
        Display a yellow indicator
    Else If the medication was due an hour or more ago then
        Display a red indicator
    Else
        Display a green indicator
Iteration (loop):
    Until the patient is discharged
        Determine if medication is due for the patient
    End Until

3. Entities

An **entity** is a person, place, thing, or event. An entity type is a collection of entity instances such as patients. An entity instance is information about an entity—one patient such as Bob Smith. The goal of the clinical systems analyst is to identify information for all clinical processes in a clinical system by identifying entities and relationships among entities commonly called **entity relationships** (Figure 2–4).

Relationships among these entities are:

- A patient has a practitioner.

- A patient has a nurse.

- A practitioner writes medical orders.

- A nurse carries out medical orders.

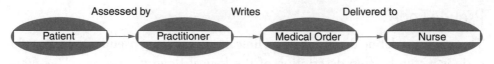

FIGURE 2–4 • Entities are people or things such as a patient, practitioner, nurse, and medical order. Relationships define the relation among entities.

- A practitioner writes medication orders.
- The nurse administers medication to the patient.

Attributes

After entities are identified, focus moves to identifying **attributes** of each entity. Think of an attribute as a characteristic of an entity—information about an entity.

Here are a few attributes of the entity patient:

- Medical record number
- Visit identifier
- First name
- Middle name
- Last name
- Date of birth
- Home street
- Home city
- Home state
- Home postal code
- Home country

Naming an Attribute

Be careful when naming an attribute. The attribute name must relate to the characteristics of the attribute. The attribute name must be meaningful and self-documenting. That is, the attribute name by itself describes the attribute. The name must be unique and readable and should be a singular noun and follow a standard format. For example, an attribute called *number* doesn't tell you much. However, an attribute called *medical record number* tells you everything you need to know about that attribute.

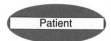

Patient Number : **15432**	Patient Home Street : **555 South Street**
Patient First Name : **Mary**	Patient Home City : **New York City**
Patient Middle Name : **Ann**	Patient Home State : **NY**
Patient Last Name : **Jones**	Patient Home Zip : **10012**

FIGURE 2–5 • An instance of an entity contains real information about the entity such as patient information.

Define each attribute as required or optional. A required attribute means the attribute must have a value for every entity instance such as a medical record number. Optional attribute means that a value is not necessary for the attribute such as the patient's middle name.

> **NURSING ALERT**
>
> Always review instances of an entity to determine what the information looks like (Figure 2–5). This is commonly referred to as an attribute instance. An attribute instance is real information of an attribute. This will help you later further define an attribute.

Composite Attributes

Be alert for composite attributes. A composite attribute is an attribute that has meaningful component parts. That is, a composite attribute is composed of simple attributes. The goal is to decompose a composite attribute into its simple attributes.

For example, a patient's home address is a composite attribute that can be broken down into elements of the address. Only simple attributes are stored in the database, All composite attributes must be reduced to simple attributes.

Single or Multiple Values

Next identify if a simple attribute can have a single or multiple values. A single value occurs when the attribute can have only one value. A multi-valued attribute can take on more than one value for an entity instance.

For example, the attribute medical record number can have one value per patient—a medical record number. However, the patient's practitioner's attribute can have multiple values. That is, more than one practitioner can be caring for the patient.

Derived Attributes

Some attributes are derived from other attributes. A derived attribute has a value that can be calculated from related attribute values. As a general rule, a derived attribute is not stored in a database because it unnecessarily takes up space. Derived attributes are calculated whenever requested.

For example, the patient's age attribute is derived from the patient's date of birth attribute and the current date attribute. That is, subtracting the patient's date of birth from the current date will result in the patient's age.

Valid Values

Next determine if an attribute must have a specific value commonly referred to as a valid value. Valid values of attributes are values that can be assigned to an attribute. An invalid value is automatically rejected by the database management system (DBMS).

Here a student number must have a fixed number of digits. For example, a visit identifier is a 12-digit number in some healthcare facilities; therefore, the visit identifier attribute must have 12 digits. Fewer than or more than 12 digits will cause the DBMS to reject the value. Only a valid medical record number is acceptable. You must determine if an attribute requires valid values and what those values are.

Entity Relationships

An entity relationship is the association between two or more entities such as a patient having many medication orders. The term *cardinality of relationships* is used to describe the relationship between entities.

There are four common relationships:

- One-to-one relationship: This type of relationship has an equal number of entities. Each patient has one home address.
- One-to-many relationship: In this type of relationship, one entity is related to many entities. A patient can have many medication orders.
- Many-to-one relationship: There are many patients who have the same practitioner.

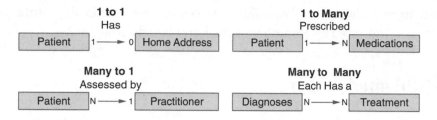

FIGURE 2–6 • Cardinality constraint identifies the number of instance in relationships of entities. Here a zero cardinality means a patient may be homeless or will have a home.

- Many-to-many relationship: A patient can have many diagnosis and many treatments.

Cardinality constraint is a term used to describe the number of instances in the relationships between entities (Figure 2–6).

- A zero value means there can be a patient who may not have a medication order. The relationship is considered optional.

- A 1 or more value means at least one relationship exists such as every medication order has a patient.

- A maximum cardinality is when there is a limit set in the relationship such as each room on the unit can have no more than two patients.

Primary Key

You must come up with a unique way to identify each instance of an entity. The identifier is referred to as **primary key**. The value of the primary key will not change in value and must have a value. For example, a medical record number and the visit identifier is an ideal identifier for each patient.

Entity Notation

Entity notation is used to depict the data model for your database. Each entity is identified in a box with the name of the entity at the top of the box. The first row within the box is the name of the attribute that uniquely identifies the instance of the entity which is called the primary key.

You can insert subsequent columns to the right of the attribute name to indicate:

- Required or optional
- Derived value (one that is calculated)
- Valid values

An arrow indicates a relationship between entities. Cardinality of the relationship is indicated by a number or the letter N indicating many.

4. Object-Oriented Design

Object-oriented design uses a natural approach to designing a clinical system. We naturally see things as objects such as a car. An **object** has attributes or information. Mention a car and you may think of make, model, color, and other features, which are all attributes. An object has behaviors. A car goes forward and backward, the car stops, and the headlights go on and off—all of these are behaviors of a car.

An object is very similar to an entity because both have attributes. However, an object also has behaviors (Figure 2–7). A behavior is a thing that the object can do, commonly referred to as a **method**, operation, or a service. We'll call behavior a method. Combining attributes and behaviors in an object is called encapsulation, which is the way we naturally view things.

Here are four methods for a patient:

- A patient can be admitted to the healthcare facility.
- A patient can accept treatment.
- A patient can refuse treatment.
- A patient can be discharged from the healthcare facility.

A behavior is a process that is identified in the leveling diagram. A behavior is described in pseudo code.

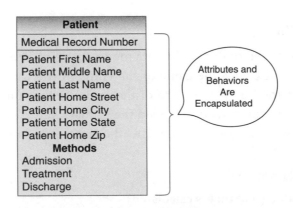

FIGURE 2−7 • An object called patient that is uniquely identified by the medical record number and contains both attributes (data) and methods (functionality).

Here is an example of pseudo code for treatment:

The patient is offered treatment by the nurse
If the patient accepts treatment then
    The nurse performs the treatment
    The nurse documents that the treatment was performed
    Reassesses the patient within an hour to determine if there were any
    side effects to the treatment
    The nurse documents the reassessment
Else
    Treatment is not performed
    The nurse documents that the patient refused treatment
    The nurse notifies the practitioner that the patient refused treatment
End If

An object can call methods of other objects by sending the method a message. A message is similar to a text message except the message usually contains a few words. The message is used by the method to perform a behavior.

For example, an object called Room Manager manages all rooms in the healthcare facility. A method of the Room Manager is to Book A Room. The Book A Room method looks like this:

Book A Room (Room ID, Requestor Name, Date/Time Requested)
Look up Room ID
If Room ID found then
    Determine if Date/Time Requested available
    If Date/Time Requested is available then
        Assign Requestor Name to the room
        Return message "Room has successfully been booked."
    Else
        Return message "Room is unavailable"
    End IF
Else
    Return message "Room ID not found"
End IF

This method refers to the message—commonly referred to as reading the message—and then uses the content of the message for processing. The message consists of three pieces of information. These are the Room ID, Requestor Name, and Date/Time Requested. Based on the content of the message, the method books the room. You'll notice that the method sends a return message to the object that called the method indicating if the room was successfully booked or not.

For example, the admissions department can call this method on behalf of the patient to book a room on a unit. Likewise, a surgeon can call this object to book an operating room. Here is the pseudo code that calls the method:

Book A Room (A2201, MR12345, 8/28/14)

NURSING ALERT

A case narrative tool is useful to help identify objects in a clinical system. A number of case narrative tools are available in the marketplace.

---

5. Data Capture

Data capture is the identification and acquisition of new data at the source of the data, which is usually data entry but can also be electronic data transferred from another computing device. Data entry is the process of translating the source data into a computer readable format and occurs by using a data input device such as the keyboard, mouse, touch screens, bar code reader, smart cards, or a biometric reader. The systems analyst decides on the data input device and the programmer incorporates the input device into the system.

NURSING ALERT

As a rule of thumb, keep the number of clicks to perform a task to the minimum to make the data capture efficient.

The screen is the face of the application, and its design determines the application's success. A well-designed screen should:

- Only capture data that cannot be calculated or looked up. This is called variable data.
- Highlight errors on the screen so the user can easily see and fix the problem such as undo a task.
- Use a menu bar containing common functions that can be quickly selected.
- Enable shortcuts to functions such as a right click popup menu.
- Provide navigational and procedural help, including where to find something and how to do something.

- The flow of data entry should be logical.
- Make the screen appear similar to the paper form currently in use. This is referred to as a metaphor for a screen and reduces the need for training. Users can intuitively navigate the screen because the screen design is familiar.
- Use appropriate graphical user interface controls for data entry. Most controls are familiar.
- Validate all data, if possible.
- Make sure required data is entered.
- Enforce data format.
- Make sure that data makes sense by checking for an acceptable data range. For example, a practitioner may order a blood glucose finger stick four times a day. The clinical system should ask the practitioner to confirm a request to check blood glucose more frequently.

> **NURSING ALERT**
>
> Create a prototype of each screen. A prototype is a simulation of screens. Let users interact with screens. Encourage them to recommend improvement and then incorporate recommendations into the system.

6. Application Architecture

Application architecture is technologies used to implement the information systems. For example, a system might reside on a central computer called a server. The system is accessed by other computers referred to as clients. This is referred to as the application's architecture.

A clinical information system has three components:

- The application program, which is the logic of the application.
- The DBMS that manages the database.
- The database

Local application architecture is one where all three components reside on the same computer. An advantage is speed because all operations occur on one computer and only one computer needs to be upgraded when a component changes. A major disadvantage is the application and the data cannot easily be shared with other users.

Modern application architecture divides an information system into five components referred to as layers. These are:

- The presentation layer: This is the user interface.
- The presentation logic layer: This is the piece that generates the presentation layer.
- The application logic layer: This is where clinical rules and data are processed.
- The data manipulation layer: This contains software that interacts with the database.
- The data layer: This is where the data resides.

Each component is positioned in the appropriate place in the architecture to deliver the most effective response to users.

File Server Architecture

File server architecture is one of the first type of information system architecture and is still used today. A file server is a computer that stores and serves up files. Think of a file server as a shared hard disk. Computers and the file server are connected to a local area network, which is used to transfer files to and from the file server.

The advantage is that files can be shared among computers. A major disadvantage is that the data stored in those files is not managed.

A file can be copied to one or more computers, and each computer can change the content of the file, resulting in subsequent files overwriting files stored on the file server. Changes to the file are lost except for those made by the last computer saving the file.

Client/Server Architecture

Client/server architecture is a major improvement over file server architecture. The presentation logic layer and application layer are on the client. The data manipulation layer and the database are on the server.

These are referred to as **tiers**, and the architecture is referred to as a two-tier architecture.

- Tier 1 contains front-end functions at the client.
- Tier 2 contains back-end functions at the server.

Client/server architecture is also commonly known as fat client because each client has application software running on it. Application software must be reinstalled on every computer—client—when the software changes. This is a challenge for large corporations that require updating of thousands of computers in a short time period.

Thin Client Application Architecture

A **thin client** application architecture is where no application software runs on clients and is referred to as three-tier architecture. The advantages of three-tier architecture are that the application resides in one place, and upgrades occur on one computer.

- Tier 1 is the client layer: The client accesses the application from the application server.
- Tier 2 is the business layer: The application resides on an application server.
- Tier 3 is the database layer: This contains the DBMS and the database.

Internet Architecture

Internet architecture is the architecture used by Internet and intranet applications and is a multi-tier architecture.

- Tier 1 is the client: The client accesses the system using a browser.
- Tier 2 is the web server: The web server sends the client a webpage.
- Tier 3 is the application server: The application sever contains the application. Common gateway interface (CGI) programs on the web server interact with applications on the application server.
- Tier 4 is the database layer: This is where the DBMS and database reside.

Initially, the client uses the browser to request a web page known as the home page. Users input data into the browser, and the browser sends a request to the web server. The web server runs a CGI program that reads the request and data and then runs the appropriate application program. The application program returns data to the CGI program, which then generates a dynamic web page that is sent to the client.

Cloud Architecture

Cloud architecture is a distribution architecture that makes files, applications, and the database available anytime from anywhere. This is an on-demand broad network that can use any distributive architecture. The advantage of cloud architecture is the availability of systems from anywhere in the world. The challenge is security.

A transaction application is one of the most common types of applications and uses a unique architecture.

Transaction Architecture

A transaction is an activity that has multiple processes such as admitting a patient to a healthcare facility. This transaction requires gathering and storing general information about the patient, insurance information, and health information as well as booking a room on a unit. The information is stored in multiple tables in the database. The transaction succeeds only if all processes involved in the transaction are successfully completed. If one process fails, then the entire transaction fails.

Scalability by Design

Scalability is the ability to increase or decrease a clinical application to match changes in demand. Let's say that a healthcare facility wants to consolidate with another healthcare facility. Rather than redesigning or purchasing a new clinical system, the healthcare facilities would increase the capacity of the current clinical system. The ability to increase capacity quickly depends on whether the current clinical system is scalable. That is, components of the clinical system can easily be replicated.

An example of scalability is used to solve a common problem with a transactional architecture. In a transactional architecture, one DBMS is used on one database server to store new transactions and used to retrieve transactional information. That is, it stores patient information and retrieves patient information.

Response time decreases when there is heavy demand on the DBMS. That is, there are many updates to patient information at the same time as there are many requests to retrieve patient information. All updates and requests for information are processed by the same DBMS on the same database server.

One method of addressing this problem is to have a mirrored database running on a different database server. As patient information is updated on the primary DBMS and database, the patient information is automatically updated on the mirrored database. All requests for patient information are handled by the mirrored database, thereby reducing demand on the primary database.

The benefit of a scalable design is realized when demand increases. The MIS department needs only to add another mirrored database to balance the demand for patient information, thereby increasing the response time for information.

CASE STUDY

CASE 1

The executive nurse of the healthcare facilities assigns you the task of designing the healthcare facility's electronic medical record systems. The electronic medical record system must be available 24/7 to 34 units throughout the facility. Each unit has one nurse's station and four COWs (computers on wheels) that are taken into each patient room during medication administration, procedures, and assessments. Each nurse's station has six computers that are shared among practitioners, unit clerks, and the nursing staff. The electronic medical record system must exchange data among the CPOE, eMAR, pharmacy, and administrative systems. The executive nurse asks you the following questions. What are your best responses?

QUESTION 1. What does scalability mean?
ANSWER: Scalability is the capability of an application to expand and contract based on a long-term change in census without the need to modify the application. This results in incremental cost increases when the application is expanded to meet new demand rather than incurring cost to acquire and Implement a new application.

QUESTION 2. How do you plan to define the needs of the healthcare facility?
ANSWER: The initial step is to begin with the whole clinical process and divide it into small processes called a work package using a technique called the work breakdown structure. Each work package is described using data flow and leveling diagrams. Details for each work package are described in English-like logic called pseudo code.

QUESTION 3. Why do you have to perform in-depth analysis if the healthcare facility is purchasing either off-the-shelf or tailored software from a vendor?
ANSWER: In-depth analysis clearly defines the clinical processes of the healthcare facility, that is, how the healthcare facility delivers healthcare to patients. Vendor software has its own workflow that may or may not conform to the healthcare facility's workflow. The in-depth analysis can be used to compare the healthcare facility's workflow with that of workflows of vendor's software. The goal is to find vendor software that compliments the healthcare facility's workflow.

QUESTION 4. Can the in-depth analysis of the healthcare facility's workflow be beneficial if the healthcare facility purchases software that can be tailored?

ANSWER: Yes. A comparison of the healthcare facility's workflow with that of the vendor software is performed to clearly identify differences. This is called a gap analysis. The vendor determines if the vendor's application can be tailored to meet the healthcare facility's workflow. If so, then the in-depth analysis serves as a map to tailor the application. If not, then administrators will know which of the healthcare facility's workflows needs to be modified.

FINAL CHECK-UP

1. **A student nurse asks you to describe a clinical information system. What is your best response?**

   A. A clinical information system is an electronic medical record system.

   B. A clinical information system is data that is processed, stored, and used to care for a patient.

   C. A clinical information system is patient information stored in a database.

   D. A clinical information system consists of patients and the patients' medical teams, data that is collected, processed, stored, and provided as output needed to care for a patients.

2. **Who is a stakeholder?**

   A. A stakeholder is any patient who has an interest in an existing or proposed clinical information system.

   B. A stakeholder is any person who has an interest in an existing or proposed clinical information system.

   C. A stakeholder is any clinician who has an interest in an existing or proposed clinical information system.

   D. A stakeholder is any administrator who has an interest in an existing or proposed clinical information system.

3. **Who arranges funding for the clinical system and determines what the system will do?**

   A. System owner

   B. Project manager

   C. Stakeholder

   D. Programmer

4. **What is the role of a clinical systems analyst?**

   A. Manages the financial aspects of the clinical system.

   B. Develops the systems from specifications provided by stakeholders and clinicians who are going to use the clinical system.

   C. Manages the clinical system project.

   D. Identifies the clinical requirements of the clinical system and translates clinical requirements into clinical specifications for the system.

5. **What is the definition of work breakdown structure?**

   A. Dividing tasks among resources.

   B. A process of decomposing a simple request into smaller and smaller components that are easy to comprehend and analyze.

   C. A process of creating a complex system from small components.

   D. Breaking down tasks into milestones.

6. **What is the purpose of using a leveling diagram?**

   A. To describe the work breakdown structure.

   B. To better understand the workflow.

   C. To discuss elements of the system with different clinicians.

   D. A leveling diagram is a data flow diagram that gradually breaks down a process into detailed processes.

7. **What is the purpose of pseudo code?**

   A. Pseudo code is a step-by-step description of the logical flow of a process.

   B. Pseudo code decreases logical errors in the system.

   C. Pseudo code increases steps in the logical flow of a process.

   D. Pseudo code decreases steps in the logical flow of a process.

8. **What is the purpose of a primary key?**

   A. A primary key uniquely identifies each instance of an attribute.

   B. A primary key uniquely identifies all instances of an attribute.

   C. A primary key uniquely identifies all instances of an entity.

   D. A primary key uniquely identifies each instance of an entity.

9. **What is a method of an object?**

   A. A method is used to define an object.

   B. A method is a behavior of an object.

   C. A method is used to define an attribute.

   D. A method is used to define an entity.

10. **How would you measure the efficiency of data capture?**
    A. Let a clinical systems designer design data capture without input from stakeholders.
    B. Let stakeholders design the system.
    C. Keep the number of clicks to perform a task to the minimum.
    D. Let a clinical systems designer design data capture with input from stakeholders.

CORRECT ANSWERS AND RATIONALES

1. D. A clinical information system is an arrangement of patients and the patient's medical team, data, processes, and information technology that interact to collect, process, store, and provide as output the information needed to care for a patient.
2. A. A stakeholder is any patient who has an interest in an existing or proposed clinical information system.
3. A. System owner
4. D. Identifies the clinical requirements of the clinical system and translates clinical requirements into clinical specifications for the system.
5. B. A process of decomposing a simple request into smaller and smaller components that are easy to comprehend and analyze.
6. D. A leveling diagram is a data flow diagram that gradually breaks down a process into detailed processes.
7. B. Pseudo code decreases logical errors in the system.
8. D. A primary key uniquely identifies each instance of an entity.
9. B. A method is a behavior of an object.
10. C. Keep the number of clicks to perform a task to the minimum.

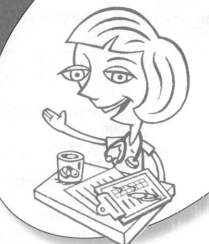

chapter 3

Clinical Database Analysis

KEY TERMS

Clinical database application	Logical database design
Data	Normalization
Data modeling	Physical database design
Database	Query
Database Management System (DBMS)	Referential integrity
Entities	Relational database
Entity attribute	Structured data
Entity instance	Structured Query Language (SQL)
Entity type	Unstructured data
Index	User interface

1. Clinical Database Application

A **clinical database application** is a computer program that is used to store and retrieve patient information or information necessary for patient care. Commonly used clinical database applications include an electronic medical record, an electronic medical administration record, a computer physician order enter system, and an order management system.

A clinical database application consists of a:

- **User interface**: A user interface is a computer program that enables the clinician to store, retrieve, edit, and delete clinical information.

- **Database Management System (DBMS)**: A DBMS is a computer application that manages information stored in the database.

- **Database**: A database is an electronic filing cabinet that contains clinical information.

The user interface is the portion of the clinical database application that you can see. You cannot see DBMS, database and information stored in the database because these are in a remote location connected to your computer by a computer network.

> **NURSING ALERT**
>
> Clinical information is never deleted. Instead, the information is marked as strike and amended, indicating that the information was corrected. The incorrect information remains but is not active.

A clinician enters request for information into the user interface. The request is sent to the DBMS, where the request is processed, and information is returned and displayed on the computer screen by the user interface. For example, a nurse requests a list of patients who are on the nurse's unit by entering the unit's name into the user interface. The DBMS searches the database for patients on the specified unit and returns information about those patients to the user interface where the information is displayed on the computer screen.

How the Clinical Database Application Is Developed

A systems analyst assesses the clinical needs and translates those needs into specifications for the clinical application. A database analyst or designer translates identified information required by the clinical application specifications into **data** and into a database design called a database schema.

Think of information as a group that provides meaning to the data. For example, a patient's medical record number, visit identifier, and name are information that describes a patient. A database designer reduces information to data. Data is stored in a database. Patient data is:

- Medical record number
- Visit identifier
- First name
- Middle name
- Last name

There are two general categories of data:

- **Unstructured data**: images, video, audio, scanned documents
- **Structured data**: numbers, text, dates

Entities

A database analyst or designer begins to design a database schema by identifying **entities** associated with the clinical database application. An entity is a person, place, thing, or event. For example, a patient is an entity, an order is an entity, and a medication is an entity.

An entity is identified by:

- **Entity type**: An entity type is a category of entity such as patient, order, or medication.
- **Entity attribute**: An entity attribute is a characteristic of an entity such as patient medical record number, patient visit identifier, patient first name,

patient middle name, and patient last name. An entity attribute is usually data associated with an entity type.

- **Entity instance**: An entity instance is data associated with a real entity. For example, values of an entity attribute such as MR#12345, Visit ID 300001234, or Mary Margaret Jones.

Data and Database

Data is a component of information that is organized into a database. A database is an organized collection of logically related data. In this example, a patient is represented by information.

Data associated with a patient is:

- Patient information
- Diagnoses information
- Treatment information
- Billing information

Data are logically grouped together based on their relationships—patient, diagnoses, treatment, and billing.

Spreadsheet and Database

Think of a database as an Excel Workbook. Keep a workbook in mind when thinking about how a database is organized.

- A workbook typically contains information about a process. A workbook is divided into:
  - Tables similar to tables of a database.
- Each table contains data about an entity.
  - A table in an excel workbook is divided into columns and rows similar to a table in a database.
- A column contains attributes about an entity type.
- A row contains an entity instance—an actual patient.

Creating a Database

DBMS software is used to create, maintain, and provide controlled access to the database. MySQL, Oracle, SQL Server by Microsoft, DB2 by IBM, and Sybase are popular DBMS.

> ## NURSING ALERT
>
> Microsoft Access is another DBMS software, although it is less robust than others.

Requests are made to the DBMS using a **query** that is written using **Structured Query Language (SQL)**. A query is similar to a message sent to the DBMS telling the software to do something such as retrieve information.

An interactive user interface is available for many DBMS, enabling the user to use drop-down lists and other graphical user interface conventions to enter search criteria. The user interface generates the query and sends the query to the DBMS.

Most queries are embedded in a database application using an application programming interface (API). An API is a tool available to programmers enabling them to access a database from within their program.

In a clinical database application, the application user interface gathers requests from the clinician and then generates a query and sends it to the DBMS. Part of the query is the clinician's login information that is authenticated by the DBMS before the query is processed. If the clinician is not authorized to access information, then the DBMS sends notice of the failed login to the clinical database application. The clinical database application then tells the clinician that he or she is not authorized to access the information.

The DBMS and the database are typically located on a database server. A database server is a computer connected to a network enabling computers throughout the healthcare facility—and even those outside the healthcare facility—to access the database.

2. Clinical Logical Database Design

Data modeling is a method used to define data requirements of a clinical process and identifies relationship between data elements. Data modeling begins by reviewing entities and related attributes of the clinical entity (see Chapter 2). After the data model has been defined, focus is moved to developing the clinical **logical database design**.

A clinical database uses a **relational database** design in which data is organized efficiently for speedy retrieval, integrity of the data, and storage space. In a relational database design, most duplicate information is removed from the database. The single instance of the data is placed in a table within the database and is referenced each time the information is needed.

Let's take a look at a medication order to see how a relational database is organized. The following information is associated with a medication order:

- Patient electronic medical record number
- Patient visit identifier
- Patient name
- Patient location
- Patient allergies
- Order number
- Generic medication name
- Brand medication name
- Dose
- Route
- Time
- Parameters
- Practitioner writing the order

Imagine the space required to store 10 medication orders for one patient and then assume there are thousands of patients each year in the healthcare facility. Electronic storage is significant. However, a relational database design reduces storage space significantly. Here's how this is done.

In this example, the following patient information is duplicated for each order.

- Patient electronic medical record number
- Patient visit identifier
- Patient name
- Patient location
- Patient allergies

We can place this information into its own table and uniquely identify this by a combination of the patient electronic medical record number and the patient visit identifier. The patient electronic medical record number combined with the patient visit identifier will be used to identify the patient information. This is the primary key for the patient.

Likewise, the medication's generic name and brand name along with other information about the medication can be placed in its own table and uniquely identified by a medication number. This is the primary key for the medication.

Order information can also be placed in its own table identified uniquely by the order number. The order number is the primary key.

The entry in the order table will contain order information. Instead of the patient information and medication information, the order table will contain the patient's medical records number and visit identifier and the medication number.

When the order is referenced, the DBMS retrieves patient information using the patient information and medication information using the medication number.

Relational Database

A relational database is appreciably smaller in size than a corresponding flat database because duplicate data is removed. A relation is a named, two-dimensional table of data consisting of rows and columns.

To qualify as a relation, the relation must have:

- A unique name.
- Attributes with a single value.
- Each row unique. No two rows can have the same value.
- A unique name for each column. The order of columns and rows is irrelevant.
- A primary key. A primary key is a unique identifier of the relation such as patient medical record number and visit identifier.
- A foreign key. A foreign key is a primary key of another table and is used to define a dependent relation (Figure 3–1).

Parent Relation

A parent relation occurs when information in a table depends on the existence of data in another table. For example, the patient information table and the order table have a parent relation. That is, an entry in the order table must have a related entry in the patient information table. No order can exist without a patient.

Referential Integrity

Referential integrity is critical to a relational database. Without it, tables could not be logically linked together. Referential integrity occurs when a foreign key value matches a primary key value in a relation. That is, the patient medical

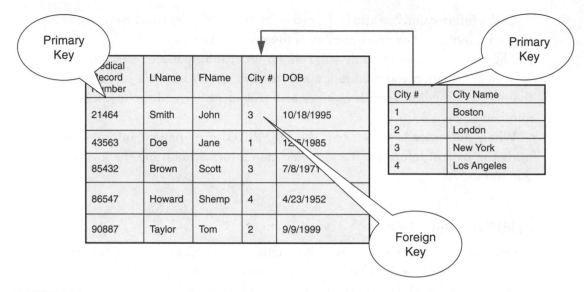

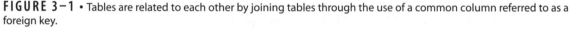

FIGURE 3–1 • Tables are related to each other by joining tables through the use of a common column referred to as a foreign key.

record number and visit identifier in the order table—which is a foreign key—matches a patient medical record number and visit identifier in the patient information table.

Delete Rules

Deleting information in a clinical database must follow referential integrity rules to prevent violating referential integrity. Here are the delete rules:

- Restrict delete rule: The restrict delete rule states that no parent side information in a parent table (row) can be deleted unless all corresponding rows in children tables are also deleted. That is, if a patient is removed from the patient information table, then all orders for the patient's medical record number and visit identifier must also be removed.

- The cascade delete rule: The cascade delete rule states that parent information and corresponding children information must be deleted automatically when the parent information is deleted.

Translate Entities to the Logical Database Design

Translating entities to the logical database design is referred to as mapping an entity to a table (Figure 3–2). You can do this by placing attribute names in a box and placing each box end to end—similar to column names.

Entity

> **Patient**
> Medical Record Number
> Patient First Name
> Patient Last Name
> Patient Street
> Patient City
> Patient State
> Patient Zip

Table

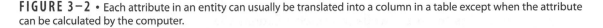

Medical Record Number	Patient First Name	Patient Last Name	Patient Street	Patient City	Patient State	Patient Zip

FIGURE 3–2 • Each attribute in an entity can usually be translated into a column in a table except when the attribute can be calculated by the computer.

You may come across a multi-value attribute. That is an attribute that has more than one value. You cannot place a multi-value attribute in a table with other attributes of the entity. Instead, create a new table for the multi-value attribute and relate the table to the entity using a foreign key.

Mapping one-to-many relationships to a logical database design is also done by using multiple tables.

For example, a patient may have more than one order; therefore, patient information and order information are placed in separate tables and are related by the patient medical record number and visit identifier.

> **NURSING ALERT**
>
> A clinical process can require complex relationships. It is important that you take time to carefully translate the data model of a process to the logical database design using the techniques shown here. Do not rush your analysis. Your logical database design becomes the foundation for developing the actual database.

Normalization

The process of removing duplicate data is called **normalization**. There are situations when some data is duplicated, but these are very few instances. Whenever you see the same data being stored in multiple tables, create another table and relate both tables using a foreign key.

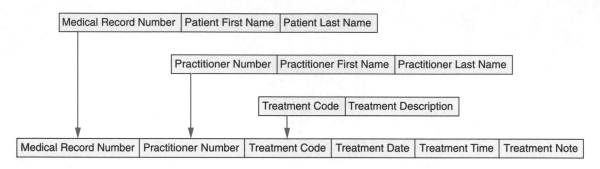

FIGURE 3–3 • Normalization enables the mapping of complex relationships to tables in a database as illustrated by creating a treatment table.

The goal is to create well-structured relations that contain minimal data redundancy and permit users to interact with the database without causing data inconsistencies when inserting, deleting, or modifying data.

The normalization process requires three steps called forms.

- First normal form: Remove multi-valued attributes by placing them in their own tables.

- Second normal form: A primary key must identify groups of non-key attribute. For example, all attributes of a patient are identified by a medical record number and visit identifier in a row of a table.

- Third normal form: The primary key must not be determined by another attribute.

At first the normalization process may seem confusing. Focus on techniques that show you how to remove duplicate data and how to uniquely identify rows using a primary key, and you will be able to develop a logical design for your database (Figure 3–3).

3. Clinical Physical Database Design

After the data model has been converted into a logical database design in which attributes are organized into relations in the form of tables, the next step in developing a database application is to create a **physical database design**. A physical database design contains technical specifications for storing data (Figure 3–4).

The process of transforming a logical database design to a physical database design is referred to as mapping. The goal of mapping is to identify and define fields of data commonly referred to as a column. A column is the smallest unit

Patient			
Medical Record Number	INTEGER	NOT NULL	Auto Generated
Patient First Name	VARCHAR(255)	NOT NULL	
Patient Last Name	VARCHAR(255)	NOT NULL	
Patient Street	VARCHAR(255)	NOT NULL	
Patient City	VARCHAR(255)	NOT NULL	
Patient State	VARCHAR(2)	NOT NULL	Valid State
Patient Zip	VARCHAR(255)	NOT NULL	Valid Zip Code

FIGURE 3–4 • The physical database design requires that you identify column names, data type of the data stored in the column, whether or not the column can remain empty, and rules to be applied to the column.

of application data recognized by system software. Think of this as a column in a spreadsheet table.

A column is defined as a data type. A data type defines the kind of data that can be stored in the column. A sample of data types is shown here; however, specific data types may be limited to a particular DBMS.

- VARCHAR(X) data type: This data type accepts variable length characters. The maximum number of characters that can be stored in this column is 255. You can specify the number of characters for the column within the parenthesis.

- Boolean data type: This data type defines a column that stores true/false or yes/no values.

- Integer data type: This data type defines a column that stores whole numbers.

- Decimal data type: This data type defines a column that stores partial numbers.

- Blob data type: This data type defines a column used to store images in a table. Actually, only the reference to the image is stored in the table. The image itself is stored elsewhere in the database.

- Text data type: This data type defines a column used to store large amount of text. This text is not searchable directly by the DBMS.

- Timestamp: This data type defines a column that stores date and time in the table. Typically, timestamp causes the DBMS to automatically enter the current date and time.

Special characteristics of an attribute value, such as being required or optional, are used to define the column description. Here are examples of column descriptions that are common to many DBMS.

- NOT NULL: This indicates that the column cannot be empty. For example, the patient medical record number column must have a value.

- Auto-generated value: This describes a column where the value is automatically entered by the DBMS such as the current date and time.

- Validate: This requires that the value entered into the column is validated based on clinical rules.

- Default value: This specifies a value that is to be entered into the column by the DBMS if no value was entered by the user of the application. For example, the state abbreviation for a patient may be default to the state where the healthcare facility is located.

- Valid range of values: This specifies a range of valid values that can be stored in a column. For example, a valid medical records number may range from 1000 to 9999.

Index

Data in a database can be located quickly if the data is indexed. A database **index** is similar to an index of a book, in that the index contains the data being searched and the location of that data in the table. You specify in your design indexes required by your database application.

The column in an index that is searched is called a key. Think of an index as a two-column table. The first column contains the data being searched such as last name. Last names are automatically alphabetized. The second column is the row number in the customers table that contains each last name. In this example, a search for "Jones" returns rows 2 and 3—Mary Jones and Joan Jones.

More than one column can be indexed. This is referred to as a cluster index. For example, an index created using last name, first name is a cluster index. Searching for Mary Jones in this example returns the second row—Mary Jones.

NURSING ALERT

Too many indexes decrease performance because each index must be updated whenever the key changes in the database.

CASE STUDY

CASE 1

The chief operating officer of the healthcare facility needs to know how the new electronic medical record systems will store and retrieve clinical information for use by clinicians and administrators. The electronic medical record system is provided by a vendor and tailored to complement the workflow of the healthcare facility. Practitioners will have access to the system from inside and outside the healthcare facility. The chief operating officer has general knowledge of computing but wants to know the facts about the clinical database used by the electronic medical records system. She asks the following questions. What is the best response?

QUESTION 1. Can clinical information be deleted from the database?
ANSWER: Technically, clinical information can be deleted from the database; however, the electronic medical record system only permits authorized staff to strike and amend erroneous clinical information rather than delete the clinical information. The clinical information that was stricken remains in the clinical database marked as being in error. This enables auditors to follow the trail of documentation.

QUESTION 2. How can the electronic medical record system enforce health insurance portability and accountability act (HIPAA) regulations?
ANSWER: Authorization to interact with specific patient information is assigned to the staff member's ID, enabling the DBMS to limit access to authorized information. Furthermore, each staff member's activity in the DBMS is recorded in a log that can be audited if HIPAA violations are suspected.

QUESTION 3. How can the staff share the clinical database?
ANSWER: The clinical database is managed by a DBMS. Both the DBMS and the database are stored on a database server, which is a powerful computer. The database server is connected to the healthcare facility's computer network. Any staff member who has access to the healthcare facility's network and authorization to access the clinical database can access the DBMS by making requests over the healthcare facility's network to the database server.

QUESTION 4. Will the nurse informatics specialist or the MIS department create the clinical database?
ANSWER: No. The DBMS and database are installed by the vendor as part of the vendor's electronic medical record application. The healthcare facility's staff uses the vendor's electronic medical record application to interact with the database. A programmer in the MIS department may have limited direct access to the DBMS to create management reports depending on the licensing arrangement with the vendor.

FINAL CHECK-UP

1. **What is a clinical database?**

   A. A clinical database is the electronic repository of patient information or information necessary for patient care.

   B. A clinical database is a computer program that is used to store and retrieve patient information or information necessary for patient care.

   C. A clinical database is a computer application that is used to store and retrieve patient information or information necessary for patient care.

   D. A clinical database is a database server used to store clinical information.

2. **What is a DBMS?**

   A. A DBMS is a computer application that manages access to clinical information stored in several database applications.

   B. A DBMS is a computer application that merges information stored in several database applications.

   C. A DBMS is a computer application that manages information stored in the database.

   D. A DBMS is a computer application that gives patients access to their clinical information admissions information from home.

3. **What is an instance of an entity?**

   A. An instance of an entity consists of columns.

   B. An instance of an entity consists of rows and columns.

   C. An instance of an entity is a collection of patient information.

   D. An instance of an entity is data associated with the entity.

4. **What is a database server?**

   A. A database server is a DBMS used to store patient information.

   B. A database server is a computer connected to a network enabling computers throughout the healthcare facility to access the database.

   C. A database server is a network connection enabling computers throughout the healthcare facility to access the database.

   D. A database server is a network connection enabling computers outside the healthcare facility to access the database.

5. **What is a key feature of a relational database design?**

   A. In a relational database design, only authorized staff is able to access clinical information.

   B. In a relational database design, all conflicts with clinical information are resolved before the information is stored in the database.

   C. In a relational database design, clinical information can be stored in multiple databases.

   D. In a relational database design, most duplicate information is removed from the database.

6. **What is data modeling?**
   A. Data modeling is a method used to define data requirements of a clinical process and identifies relationship between data elements.
   B. Data modeling is a method used to design the data input for a clinical database application.
   C. Data modeling is a method used to design the data output for a clinical database application.
   D. Data modeling is a method used to design the data output and input for a clinical database application.

7. **What is a foreign key?**
   A. A foreign key is a primary key of another table and is used to define an independent clinical relationship among data.
   B. A foreign key is a primary key of another table and is used to define an independent relationship among data.
   C. A foreign key is a foreign key of another table and is used to define a dependent relation.
   D. A foreign key is a primary key of another table and is used to define a dependent relation.

8. **What is referential integrity?**
   A. Referential integrity occurs when a foreign key value is similar to a primary key value in a relation.
   B. Referential integrity occurs when a foreign key value does not match a primary key value in a relation.
   C. Referential integrity occurs when a foreign key value matches a primary key value in a relation.
   D. Referential integrity occurs when a foreign key value is substantially different than a primary key value in a relation.

9. **What is normalization?**
   A. Normalization is the process of removing duplicate data in a database design.
   B. Normalization is the process of duplicating data in a database design.
   C. Normalization is the process of developing indexes in a database design.
   D. Normalization is the process of balancing data in a database design.

10. **What is a physical database design?**
    A. A physical database design contains technical specifications for storing data.
    B. A physical database design contains technical specifications for linking data.
    C. A physical database design contains technical specifications for linking tables.
    D. A physical database design contains technical specifications for storing indexes.

CORRECT ANSWERS AND RATIONALES

1. A. A clinical database is the electronic repository of patient information or information necessary for patient care.
2. C. A DBMS is a computer application that manages information stored in the database.
3. D. An instance of an entity is data associated with the entity.
4. B. A database server is a computer connected to a network enabling computers throughout the healthcare facility to access the database.
5. D. In a relational database design, most duplicate information is removed from the database.
6. A. Data modeling is a method used to define data requirements of a clinical process and identifies relationship between data elements.
7. D. A foreign key is a primary key of another table and is used to define a dependent relation.
8. C. Referential integrity occurs when a foreign key value matches a primary key value in a relation.
9. A. Normalization is the process of removing duplicate data in a database design.
10. A. A physical database design contains technical specifications for storing data.

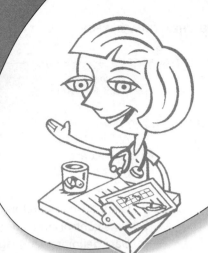

chapter 4

Clinical Data Reporting

LEARNING OBJECTIVES

1. Reporting language
2. SQL
3. Insert and retrieve information
4. Update and delete
5. Column functions
6. Group queries
7. Sorting
8. Joins
9. Transactional application
10. SQL security
11. Stored procedures

KEY TERMS

Alias	HAVING clause
ALTER clause	Index
CamelCase	Left outer join
CHECK clause	Outer join
Column	Pattern matching
Comparison operators	Query
Data control language (DCL)	Right outer join
Data definition language (DDL)	Row
Data manipulation language (DML)	SQL console
Database	Stored procedure
Database management system	Structured query language (SQL)
(DBMS)	Subquery
DISTINCT clause	Table
DROP statement	Transaction
FOR Clause	Trigger
GRANT statement	VALUES clause
GROUP BY clause	View

1. Reporting Language

Clinical applications developed by third parties have built-in reports available from within the application. The clinician can select the built-in report and specify filtering criteria that removes all but selected information from the report. The report itself is designed by the clinical software vendor and cannot be modified by the clinician.

Some third-party vendors permit the healthcare facility's management information systems (MIS) department access to the clinical **database**, enabling the clinical analyst to create custom reports using either a report writing tool such as Crystal Report or by using **Structured query language (SQL)** to retrieve clinical information from the database.

A report writing tool is a computer application that enables the clinical analyst to generate a report by using the report writing tool's user interface. The report writing tool then interacts with the clinical database to retrieve clinical information and format the clinical information into the report format designed by the clinical analyst.

In contrast, SQL is not a computer application. Rather, it is a type of programming language specifically designed to interact with the **database management system (DBMS)** to retrieve and manipulate information in the clinical database. SQL is the database language used by clinical software to interact with the clinical database. A clinical analyst who is familiar with SQL and has rights to interact with the DBMS can use SQL to generate reports and to manipulate the clinical database directly without having to use the clinical application.

NURSING ALERT

Third-party clinical software vendors may grant limited access to retrieve clinical information using SQL; however, rights to manipulate clinical information are rarely granted. Furthermore, attempts to access clinical information without proper permission are likely to invalidate any warranty and licensing agreement.

Although many clinical software applications are licensed from third-party vendors and then tailored to the needs of the healthcare facility by the clinical analyst, a clinical analyst with a team of MIS developers may create a custom clinical database application. In Chapter 2, you learned techniques needed to translate an idea for a clinical system into clinical specifications. In Chapter 3, you learned how to translate clinical specifications into a physical data model for the clinical database. In this chapter, you will learn SQL statements that enable you to translate the physical data model into a working database. In addition, you'll learn how to store, retrieve, and manipulate information in the database.

2. Structured Query Language

Interactions with a DBMS occur by sending a **query** to the DBMS. Think of a query as a message that directs the DBMS to do something with the database. The query is written using SQL. Many DBMS provide an interactive software application that enables the clinical analyst to enter a query directly and have the results of the query displayed on the computer screen. This is referred to as an **SQL console**. Clinical applications, however, have queries integrated into the clinical application. This is referred to as an embedded query.

Many DBMS recognize standard SQL statements. This means a statement that conforms to the SQL standard is able to be used with many DBMS without modifications to the query as long as the database structure is the same among DBMS. There are exceptions, however. Some DBMS will not recognize all standard SQL statements, and other DBMS have their own version of SQL that is recognized only by that DBMS.

SQL has three elements. These are:

- **Data definition language (DDL)**: DDL consists of commands used to define a database and tables.

- **Data manipulation language (DML)**: DML consists of commands used to maintain the database and to query a database.

- **Data control language (DCL)**: DCL consists of commands that control database functions.

Naming Convention

SQL is not case sensitive. However, clinical analysts commonly write SQL statements using uppercase for SQL syntax and a naming convention referred to as **CamelCase** for non-SQL syntax such as table names and **column** names. CamelCase requires that the first letter of a name is uppercase and that the name is concatenated such as FirstName. This makes it easy to read the name.

The last few letters indicate what the name represents such as DB for database, TB for **table**, and INX for **index**. These letters are either all uppercase or all lowercase depending on the case of the previous letter. For example, in the name MedicalDB, Medical ends in a lowercase; therefore, the DB is in uppercase. In contrast, PatientMRNinx is a name of an index (see Create an Index). MRN is an abbreviation for medical record number and appears in uppercase; therefore, the inx, which is the abbreviation for index, is in lowercase.

Creating a Database

A database is an electronic filing cabinet that contains clinical information. Think of a DBMS as a file clerk who maintains information in the filing cabinet. Before you can have the file clerk store information, you must first create the database (filing cabinet).

The database is created by writing an SQL query. The query consists of one statement. A statement is similar to a sentence in English. The statement contains SQL syntax and information needed by the statement. SQL syntax is words that the DBMS understands. In this example, the syntax is CREATE DATABASE, which is followed by the name we are giving to the database.

The statement ends with a semicolon. The database name should represent the nature of the database, which in this example is a medical database.

Here is the query:

CREATE DATABASE MedicalDB;

Creating a Table

After the database has been created, other SQL statements can be used to create tables for the database. Think of a table as a file folder placed in the filing cabinet. The physical database design (see Chapter 3) is translated into SQL statements that create the table.

The SQL syntax for creating a table is CREATE TABLE followed by the name of the table. The name of the table is followed by parenthesis. Within the parenthesis is the table definition. The table definition consists of one or more column definitions each separated by a comma. A column definition consists of a column name followed by the data type and attribute value (see Chapter 3). A data type (see Table 4–1) tells the DBMS the kind of data that will be stored in the column. You should define a primary key for each table (see Chapter 3).

TABLE 4–1 Common SQL Data Types	
Date Type	**Description**
CHAR (len)	Fixed length character string
CHARCTER(len)	Fixed length character string
VARCHAR(len)	Variable length character string
CHAR VARYING (len)	Variable length character string
CHARACTER VARYING (len)	Variable length character string
INTEGER	Integer number
INT	Integer number
NUMERIC (precision, scale)	Decimal numbers
DECIMAL (precision, scale)	Decimal numbers
DEC (precision, scale)	Decimal numbers
FLOAT (precision)	Floating point numbers
DATE	Calendar date
TIME(precision)	Clock time
TIMESTAMP (precision)	Date and time
MONEY	Currency

A primary key consists of values in one or more columns that uniquely identify each **row** in the table. A primary key is defined by using PRIMARY KEY followed by the column name within parentheses.

The following is the query that creates a table called patientTB. This table contains general information about a patient. You can expand upon this definition by adding additional columns to the query. Notice that the patient medical record number (patientMRN) is the primary key for this table. The NOT NULL attribute value is used to tell the DBMS that a value must be entered in each column.

```
CREATE  TABLE PatientTB (
   PatientMRN  INTEGER NOT NULL,
   PatientFirstName VARCHAR (30) NOT NULL,
   PatientMiddleName VARCHAR (60) NOT NULL,
   PatientLastName VARCHAR (60) NOT NULL,
   Street VARCHAR (60) NOT NULL,
   City VARCHAR (60) NOT NULL,
   State VARCHAR (2) NOT NULL,
   PostalCode VARCHAR(10) NOT NULL,
   PractitionerID INTEGER,
   PRIMARY KEY (PatientMRN)
);
```

NURSING ALERT

No spaces are permitted in the database name, table name, or column names. Each column name must be unique in the table. A semicolon must follow the closing parenthesis.

Creating a Table With a Constraint

A constraint is a restriction of information that can be stored in the database based on clinical rules. The constraint can be any logical statement that has a true or false result. The constraint is defined using the **CHECK clause** when the table is created. The CHECK clause requires you to specify the logical statement within parentheses.

In this example, we created a modest patient bill table. An actual patient bill table will have many more columns. The gross amount column contains the total bill. The net amount column contains the amount that is charged to the insurer and reflects the discount given to the insurer based on the insurer's contract with the hospital. Each insurer has a different discount. For this example, the insurer's discount is never more than 50% of the gross amount.

Therefore, a constraint is created on the NetAmount column using the CHECK clause. The logical expression defines the constraint. That is, the value in the NetAmount column should be equal to or greater than 50% of the amount in the GrossAmount column. An error will be displayed if the value of the NetAmount column is more than a 50% discount.

```
CREATE  TABLE PatientBillTB (
    PatientMRN  INTEGER NOT NULL,
    InsurerID  INTEGER,
    GrossAmount NUMERIC NOT NULL,
    NetAmount NUMERIC NOT NULL,
    CHECK (NetAmount >= (GrossAmount * .5))
};
```

Create an Alias for a Table

A table name should represent the kind of information that is stored in the table. For example, PatientTB implies that the table contains patient information. On occasion, the name of the table can be long and cumbersome to reference in SQL statements used to retrieve information or statements used to manipulate information in the table.

You can create a short name for the table called an **alias**. The alias can then be used in SQL statements the same way as you would use the table name. You create an alias by using the CREATE ALIAS statement followed by the short name for the table. The **FOR clause** is used to specify the table name. After an alias is defined, you can use it just like a table name in SQL queries.

In this example, we create an alias for the PatientClinicalCarePlanTB table.

```
CREATE ALIAS PtCarePlanTB
    FOR PatientClinicalCarePlanTB ;
```

An alias can be removed by using the DROP ALIAS statement as illustrated here.

```
DROP ALIAS PtCarePlanTB;
```

Adding a Column to a Table

The **ALTER clause** is used to modify an existing table. Typically, you'll use this along with the ADD clause to insert a column to an existing table. Here we are inserting a second address line to the table. Notice in the following example that the column definition is formatted the same way as the field definition is formatted in the create table statement.

```
ALTER TABLE PatientTB
    ADD Address2 VARCHAR (60);
```

Removing a Column

A column can be removed from a table by using the DROP clause in conjunction with the ALTER TABLE clause. In this example, the Address2 column is removed from the PatientTB.

```
ALTER TABLE PatientTB
  DROP Address2;
```

> **NURSING ALERT**
>
> The column being dropped from a table cannot be the column used as a primary key for the table. Remember that the value in the column that serves as the primary key uniquely identifies rows in the table.

Removing a Table

A table can be removed from a database by using the **DROP** TABLE clause. In this example, the PatientTB is being removed from the database.

```
ALTER TABLE PatientTB
  DROP Address2;
```

Creating an Index

An index is used to quickly locate search criteria in a table similar to using an index of a book to lookup information in the book (see Chapter 3). The index contains the value of the column that is being indexed and the row number that contains the value. The value of the column is a commonly used search value such as patient medical record number.

An index is created using the CREATE INDEX statement. The CREATE INDEX statement specifies a name that you give to the index and uses the ON clause to identify the table and column of that table that will be indexed. In this example, we are creating an index

```
CREATE INDEX PatientMRNidx
  ON patientTB (PatientMRN);
```

> **NURSING ALERT**
>
> The abbreviation idx is used in the name of the index to indicate to us that the name represents an index.

More than one column can be used to create an index. This is referred to as a cluster index. A common cluster index is for patient name and is used to search for a patient when the patient's medical record number is unknown.

A clustered index is created using a statement similar to the statement used to create an index. The only difference is that more than one column name is used in the ON clause. Each column name is separated by a comma. In this example, we create a clustered index on the patient name.

Notice that we specify the last name and then the first name. This is important because the search will begin with last name and then first name. There is a lower probability that multiple patients with the same last name will be in the table compared with patients with the same first name. This makes the search for the patient quicker with lastname–first name than the firstname–last name.

> **NURSING ALERT**
>
> The DBMS concatenates column values in a clustered index. For example, Bob Smith appears as SmithBob in the index.

In this example, we formed the name of the index to imply the table and column values. The last three letters of the name indicates this is an index.

CREATE INDEX PatientLastNameFirstNameIDX
    ON PatientTB (PatientLastName, PatientFirstName);

An index can be removed by using the DROP clause in a statement similar to the statement used to remove a table. Here we are removing the PatientLastNameFirstNameIDX.

DROP INDEX PatientLastNameFirstNameIDX;

3. Insert and Retrieve Information

Data can be inserted into a table by using the INSERT INTO statement. The INSERT INTO statement requires that you specify the table name. Within parentheses are data values that will be placed into the table. Notice that each data value is separated by a comma. This tells the DBMS where each data value begins and ends. Text values including numbers that are not to be used in calculations are enclosed in single quotations. Numbers are entered without quotations. The **VALUES clause** contains the data that is going to be inserted into the table.

Here we are inserting information about a new patient into the patient table. Notice that the first example does not specify column names because the order of the values corresponds to the order of columns. The DBMS assumes that we want each value to be placed into the column.

    INSERT INTO PatientTB
        VALUES ('12345', 'Mary', 'Margret', 'Jones', '555 Maple Street', 'Any City', 'NJ', '07660');

We can specify column names in the INSERT INTO statement by placing column names with parentheses as shown here. The DBMS will place the first value specified in the VALUES clause into the first column name in the INSERT INTO statement. This enables us to insert some but not all patient information. Notice in this example that the patient does not have a middle name. Therefore, we can exclude the middle name if we specify column names in the INSERT INTO statement.

    INSERT INTO PatientTB
        (PatientMRN, PatientFirstName, PatientLastName, Street, City, State, PostalCode)
        VALUES ('12345', 'Mary', 'Jones', '555 Maple Street', 'Any City', 'NJ', '07660');

Data can be inserted from another table by using the SELECT statement as part of the INSERT INTO statement. The SELECT statement (see Retrieving Information) tells the DBMS to select specified columns from a table. An asterisk is used in the following SELECT station to indicate that all columns should be retrieved. The FROM clause identifies the table.

    Here the DBMS is asked to insert all columns and rows from the patient table into the patient backup table.

    INSERT INTO PatientBackupTB
        (PatientMRN, PatientFirstName, PatientLastName, Street, City, State, PostalCode)
        SELECT *
            FROM PatientTB;

Retrieving Information

Data is retrieved from a database using the SELECT statement. The SELECT statement lists columns to be returned from one or more tables. The FROM clause is used to specify the table. All rows of the table will be returned.

    In the next sample, we are selecting all the columns of all the rows from the patient table.

```
SELECT  PatientMRN, PatientFirstName, PatientLastName, Street, City,
State, PostalCode
   FROM PatientTB;
```

You can modify the previous example to return one or several columns by specifying those columns in the SELECT statement. The following example returns the medical record number and the patient name.

```
SELECT  PatientMRN  , PatientFirstName, PatientLastName
   FROM PatientTB;
```

The WHERE Clause

Most of the time, you should select rows and columns from a table rather than all columns and all rows. Several SQL clauses can be used with the SELECT statement to fine tune a request for data. The WHERE clause is used to specify a logical expression commonly referred to as a search criteria that limits the number of rows returned by the DBMS.

In this example, the WHERE clause is used to return the patient medical record number and name for rows where the value in the PatientLastName is Jones.

```
SELECT PatientMRN, PatientFirstName, PatientLastName
   FROM PatientTB
   WHERE PatientLastName = 'Jones';
```

Multiple conditions can be specified in the WHERE clause by using another condition separated by the AND operator. Both conditions must be true for the DBMS to return a row. The following example returns the patient medical record number from rows where both the value in the PatientLastName is Jones and the value in the PatientFirstName is Mary.

```
SELECT PatientMRN
   FROM PatientTB
   WHERE PatientLastName = 'Jones' AND PatientFirstName = 'Mary';
```

Using the OR operator in place of the AND operator tells the DBMS that return rows where either condition is true. In the previous example, the OR operator causes the DBMS to return rows that contain the first name Mary or the last name Jones.

Pattern Matching

There are times when you might be unsure of the search value. That is, you have a partial value. You can use **pattern matching** in the search criteria to ask the DBMS to return rows that contain the partial value. Pattern matching is specified by using a wild card character. These are:

- Underline (_): This represents any signal character. For example, 'J_n_s' returns any value that begins with J, ends with s, and has an n as the second character.

- %: This represents zero to any number of characters. For example, 'Jo%" returns any value that begins with the letters Jo.

Pattern matching is used with LIKE or NOT LIKE operator. The LIKE operator tells the DBMS to return rows with values like the value in the pattern matching expression. The NOT LIKE operator tells the DBMS to return rows that have values unlike the pattern matching expression. The following example tells the DBMS to return the medical record number of patients who have the last name that begins with Jo.

```
SELECT PatientMRN
FROM PatientTB
WHERE PatientLastName LIKE 'Jo%';
```

Comparison Operators

You can use **comparison operators** in the search criteria to fine tune the rows that you want returned by the DBMS. A comparison operator is typically used to set a number criteria for rows that contain number values such as returning rows where the patient's net amount is greater than $1000. Here is the WHERE clause for this search criterion: Table 4–2 contains comparison operators.

```
WHERE NetAmount > 1000;
```

TABLE 4–2 Comparison Operators	
Operator	**Description**
=	Equal to
<	Less than
>	Greater than
<=	Less than or equal to
>=	Greater than or equal to
<>	Not equal to

Searching for Empty Columns

There are times when you may want to see rows that have values missing. You can ask the DBMS to return those rows by using the IS NULL clause as part of the search criteria in the WHERE clause. The following example of a WHERE clause asks the DBMS to return rows that are missing a postal code.

WHERE PostalCode IS NULL;

Likewise, you can have the DBMS return rows that have a value in a column by using the NOT NULL clause as shown here. Rows that do not have a postal code are not returned.

WHERE PostalCode NOT NULL;

Searching for Ranges

The BETWEEN clause is used to return rows whose values fall within a specified range of values. For example, let's say you want a list of patients who were admitted to the healthcare facility between 1/1/2014 and 12/31/2014. Here's the expression in the WHERE clause.

WHERE AdmissionDate BETWEEN '1/1/2014' AND '12/31/2014';

Likewise, the NOT clause can be used to exclude a range in rows returned by the DBMS as shown here.

WHERE AdmissionDate NOT BETWEEN '1/1/2014' AND '12/31/2014';

There are occasions when you want to search for a set of values rather than a range of values. For example, you may want rows of patients who live in a specific set of postal codes. You can specify a set as criteria for the WHERE clause by using the IN clause. The IN clause contains the set of values to be searched. Here's the WHERE clause that searches for a set of postal codes.

WHERE PostCode IN ('07552', '07660');

4. Update and Delete

Values in a column can be changed by using the UPDATE statement and specifying the table name. The UPDATE statement has two clauses. The SET clause specifies the column name and the new data value. The WHERE clause specifies the row that is being updated.

In this example, the patient has a new practitioner. The practitioner is identified by the practitioner's ID number, which is the value that is being placed in the PractitionerID column. Notice that the WHERE clause identifies the row that is being updated. The row is identified by specifying the patient's medical record number as a value in the PatientMRN column.

> ### NURSING ALERT
>
> The DBMS overwrites the content of the column with the value specified in the UPDATE statement.

```
UPDATE PatientTB
   SET PractitionerID = 87654
   WHERE PatientMRN = 12345;
```

The WHERE clause is optional, although you'll probably include the WHERE clause in most of your UPDATE statement because rarely will a value be updated in all rows in the table. Excluding the WHERE clause causes the DBMS to update the specified column of all rows with the value specified in the SET clause.

Deleting a Row

A row can be removed from a table by using the DELETE FROM statement and specifying the table name. The WHERE clause is used to identify the row. In this example, we are deleting all columns associated with the patient whose medical record number is 12345.

```
DELETE FROM PatientTB
   WHERE  PatientMRN = 12345;
```

All rows can be deleted from a table by using the DELETE FROM statement and excluding the WHERE clause as shown in the following example.

```
DELETE FROM PatientTB;
```

5. Column Functions

As you will recall from Chapters 2 and 4, an attribute can be derived from other attributes. For example, the patient's age can be calculated by subtracting the patient's date of birth from today's date. Data associated with a derived attribute (i.e., age) is normally not stored in the database. Instead, the data is calculated by the DBMS when data is needed to be retrieved.

SQL has functions referred to as column functions that instruct the DBMS to perform calculations. Column functions can be used in a SELECT statement

TABLE 4–3 Commonly Used Column Functions	
Calculate the Sum of Values	**Return the Lowest Value**
SELECT SUM(NetAmount) FROM PatientBillTB;	SELECT MIN(NetAmount) FROM PatientBillTB;
Count the Number of Rows that Contain Values in the Specified Column	**Return the Highest Value**
SELECT COUNT(NetAmount) FROM PatientBillTB;	SELECT MAX(NetAmount) FROM PatientBillTB;
Count the Number of Rows Regardless of Values	**Return the Average Value**
SELECT COUNT(*) FROM PatientBillTB;	SELECT AVG(NetAmount) FROM PatientBillTB;

to return the calculated value as shown in Table 4–3, which contains commonly used column functions.

Multiple column functions can be used in a SELECT statement to return different calculations by placing each column function in the SELECT statement separated by a column. This is illustrated in the next example in which we are asking the DBMS to calculate and return the minimum, maximum, and average values of the NetAmount column in the patient bill table.

    SELECT MIN(NetAmount), MAX(NetAmount), AVG(NetAmount)
        FROM PatientBillTB;

Column functions can also be used in the WHERE clause as a part of the logical expression in the selection criteria. In this example, we are asking the DBMS to calculate the average net amount, compare the average net amount with the value in the NetAmount column, and return the patient's medical record number for patients whose net amount is greater than the average net amount.

    SELECT PatientMRN
        FROM PatientBillTB
        WHERE NetAmount > AVG(NetAmount);

DISTINCT Clause

The **DISTINCT clause** removes duplicate values from the results returned by the DBMS. For example, you may need to identify practitioners who have patients currently admitted to the healthcare institution. Each practitioner is likely to have more than one patient. The PatientTB has a PractitionerID column. You can write a query asking the DBMS to return practitioner IDs for those patients. However, the returned list of practitioner IDs will likely have duplicates. You can eliminate duplicates by using the DISTINCT clause in the query. This is shown in the next example.

```
SELECT DISTINCT PractitionerID
   FROM PatientTB;
```

The DISTINCT clause can also be used in column functions. In this example, the DISTINCT clause is used to count the number of practitioners excluding duplicates.

```
SELECT COUNT(DISTINCT PractitionerID)
   FROM PatientTB;
```

6. Group Queries

The **GROUP BY clause** is used to organize return values by a column specified in the GROUP BY clause. Let's say that you want to see a list of patients organized by practitioner. The GROUP BY clause will do this for you. Here's the query.

```
SELECT PractitionerID, PatientMRN
   FROM PatientTB
GROUP BY PractitionerID;
```

The GROUP BY clause can also be used with the COMPUTE clause and a column function to calculate by grouped values. The COMPUTE clause tells the DBMS to calculate a column based on a value in another column.

For example, the patient bill table may have multiple entries of patients that reflect multiple patient visits. The GROUP BY clause combined with the COMPUTE clause can be used to total the net amount for each patient and group the result by patient medical record number.

```
SELECT PatientMRN
   FROM PatientBillTB
   GROUP BY PatientMRN
   COMPUTE SUM (NetAmount) by PatientMRN;
```

HAVING Clause

The **HAVING clause** is used to specify a criteria for a row to be included in a group. The HAVING clause parallels that of the WHERE clause, consisting of the keyword HAVING followed by a search condition. The HAVING clause specifies a search condition for groups.

The search condition in a HAVING clause can be:

- A constant
- A column function, which produces a signal value summarizing the rows in the group
- A grouping column, which by definition has the same value in every row of the group
- An expression involving combination of the above

In this example, only rows where the value of the NetAmount column is more than 10,000 will be included in the group.

```
SELECT PatientMRN
    FROM PatientBillTB
    GROUP BY PatientMRN
    HAVING NetAmount > 10000;
```

7. Sorting

The DBMS can place results in a sort order by using the ORDER BY clause. The ORDER BY clause specifies a column whose values will be sorted. Selected rows are then sorted based on the value of that column. Let's say that you want to display patient information and order the information by patient last name. Here's the query:

```
SELECT PatientMRN, PatientFirstName, PatientMiddleName,
PatientLastName
    FROM PatientTB
    ORDER BY PatientLastName;
```

NURSING ALERT

The ORDER BY clause can be used in conjunction with the GROUP BY clause to sort values by group.

8. Joins

In a relational database, data is organized in multiple tables based on the normalization rules (see Chapter 3) to reduce the amount of duplicate data stored in the database. Every row in each table is uniquely identified by a value in one or more columns, which is called a primary key (see Creating a Table).

The value of a primary key of a table can also be stored in a column of another table to link both tables. This is referred to as a foreign key. This may sound confusing; however, this example should clarify the relationship.

Let's return to the PatientTB. The primary key of the PatientTB is the patient medical record number (PatientMRN). The patient has a practitioner. The practitioner is identified in the PatientTB by the practitioner's ID number, which is stored in the PractitionerID column. The value in the PractitionerID column is a foreign key. That is, the value in the PractitionerID column is the primary key of the practitioner's table (PractitionerTB). The practitioner's table contains all the information about the practitioner.

If we wanted to retrieve patient information, we probably want to include the name of the patient's practitioner. However, the practitioner's name isn't in the patient table. It is in the practitioner's table. To retrieve the practitioner's name, we need to link the patient's row in the PatientTB with the corresponding practitioner's row in the PractitionerTB. The link is called a join—you join together two tables.

A join is made by referencing the foreign key in the PatientTB, which is the PractitionerID, to the primary key in the practitioner's table that has the same value as the foreign key in the PatientTB. The reference is made in the WHERE clause of the SQL statement by specifying the table name and the column name of two tables in the relationship.

Creating a Join

A join is created by specifying names of the tables in the FROM clause and using a logical expression in the WHERE clause to join the rows. In this example, we join the PatientTB with the PractitionerTB. Both table names are placed in the FROM clause. The WHERE clause contains the join by saying that the value of the PractitionerID in the PatientTB must equal the value of the PractitionerID in the PractitionerTB. Only those rows in both tables that match these criteria will be returned by the DBMS.

The SELECT statement contains column names of columns whose values we want to retrieve from the database. These names are of columns from both the PatientTB and from the PractitionerTB.

NURSING ALERT

You must reference the table name when using a column name only if the column name appears in both tables. When referencing the table name, the table name is separated from the column name by a period such as PatientTB.PractitionerID.

In this example, we do not have to reference the table name in the SELECT statement because each column name is unique to either the patient table or the practitioner table. However, the table name must be referenced in the WHERE clause because both the patient table and the practitioner table have a column called PractitionerID.

SELECT PatientMRN, PatientFirstName, PatientLastName, PractitionerFirstName, PractitionerLastName
   FROM PatientTB, PractitionerTB
   WHERE PatientTB.PractitionerID = PractitionerTB.PractitionerID;

> **NURSING ALERT**
>
> The join is made by the column value and not the column name. You could have different names used in each table as long as the value is the same in both tables.

Alias Table Names

A common problem that you will encounter is that the table name might be relatively long. You will notice this when referencing the table name with the column name in either the SELECT statement or in the WHERE clause. Clinical systems analysts work around this problem by declaring an alias for the table name in the FROM clause. Think of an alias as an abbreviation.

An alias can consists of one or more letters that are indicative of the table name. The alias is declared when you specify the table name in the FROM clause by placing the alias following the table name separated by a space. In this example, we use PT as the alias for PatientTB and MD for the alias for PractitionerTB. The alias is then used in expressions in place of the table name as shown here.

Notice in this example that we ask the DBMS to return the practitioner ID. Because the practitioner ID is located in both tables, we use the alias for the PractitionerTB table in the SELECT statement to reference the value of the PractitionerID column from the PractitionerTB.

SELECT PatientMRN, PatientFirstName, PatientLastName, MD.PractitionerID, PractitionerFirstName, PractitionerLastName
   FROM PatientTB PT, PractitionerTB MD
   WHERE PT.PractitionerID = MD.PractitionerID;

Outer Join

There are different types of joins each designed to address a specific circumstance of joining rows of two tables. The **outer join** is a type of join that links two tables based on matching column values in each table.

An outer join combines information from two tables by forming pairs of related rows from the two tables. The row pairs that make up the joined table are those where the matching columns in each in the two tables have the same value. The previous example that illustrated joining the patient table and the practitioner table is an example of an outer join.

Left Outer Join

A **left outer join** is another type of join. A left outer join links two tables by returning rows of the left table in the WHERE clause that match and not match of the right table. Only rows in the right table that match the left table are returned.

A left outer join combines information from two tables by forming pairs of related rows from the two tables. Matched and unmatched rows of the left table and only matched rows of the right table appear in the joined table. This can be confusing, but the next example will clarify the left outer join.

Let's say that you want returned from the database information about all visits from patients in the patient table. The patient table may contain patients who have not visited the healthcare facility. That is, they did not complete the admission process. Therefore, the patient table contains patients who have rows in the patient visit table and patients who have no records in the patient visit table.

We want to see a list of all patients regardless if they have visited the hospital, and if they did visit, we want to see their information. We need to create a left outer join to retrieve this information as shown in the next example.

The left outer join is defined by using the *= symbols in the WHERE clause expression. The join is made on the patient medical record number that appears in both the patient table and the patient visit table. We are retrieving the patient medical record number from the patient table along with the patient's name. The visit date and diagnosis are retrieved from the patient visit table. These values are empty if the patient has not visited the healthcare facility.

SELECT PT.PatientMRN, PatientFirstName, PatientLastName, VisitDate, Diagnosis
    FROM PatientTB PT, PatientVisitTB PTV
    WHERE PT.PatientMRN * = PTV.PatientMRN;

Right Outer Join

The **right outer join** is the reverse of the left outer join. That is, only rows in the left table that match rows in the right table in the WHERE clause are returned along with all the rows in the right table. The right outer join is defined using the symbol =* in the WHERE clause as shown here where we reversed the WHERE clause expression from the previous example.

    WHERE PTV.PatientMRN = * PT.PatientMRN

Subquery

A **subquery** is a query within a query. That is, there are two queries in one SQL statement, which consists of two queries. First is a subquery that asks the DBMS to retrieve a set of rows from a table. The second query (the primary query) asks the DBMS to apply the primary query to the results of the first query.

This example contains a subquery. The subquery is defined in the WHERE clause. Here we ask the DBMS to retrieve the patient medical record number from the patient bill table that has a net amount of more than $10,000. After the DBMS returns these patient medical record number, we then ask the DBMS to run the primary query that joins the patient table to the results of the subquery. That is, the patient medical record number in the returned value of the subquery is linked to the patient medical record number in the patient table. Once joined, the DBMS is asked to retrieve the patient medical record number and the patient's name.

    SELECT PatientMRN, PatientFirstName, PatientLastName
      FROM PatientTB
      WHERE PatientMRN = (SELECT PatientMRN
        FROM PatientBillTB
        WHERE NetAmount > 10000);

EXISTS

Another type of join uses the EXIST clause to determine if a value exists in another table. This is illustrated in the next example. Here we want to return the practitioner ID and practitioner name if the practitioner has a patient registered in the healthcare facility. To do this we use a subquery that selects the value of the PractitionerID column from the patient table. After these values are returned, we use the primary query to ask the DBMS to return the PractitionerID and practitioner name if the practitioner ID exists in the values returned by the subquery.

    SELECT PractitionerID, PractitionerFirstName, PractitionerLastName
      FROM PractitionerTB
      WHERE PractitionerID EXISTS (SELECT PractitionerID
        FROM PatientTB);

9. Transactional Application

A **transaction** is an interaction that may have multiple steps such as treating the patient and billing the patient for treatment. A transactional application is software that facilitates a transaction enabling each step of the transaction to be processed and stored into a database. This is referred to as a transaction processing.

Transaction processing is treated differently than simply inserting data associated with the transaction into the database. A transaction is different because each step of the transaction must succeed for the transaction to succeed. If one step fails, then the entire transaction fails.

SQL statements to process a transaction are usually embedded into an application that interacts with the person using the application. This means that the application may interact with the person during processing. The transaction can be interrupted at any point either through interaction with the user or a problem with processing. The risk is that some processing would have been completed and other processes abandoned. However, this risk is mitigated by being able to reverse processes that have been completed if other processes failed.

A transaction is created by using the START TRANSACTION statement and is followed by SQL queries for each step in the process. If the transaction is completed, then the COMMIT statement is executed, committing the transaction to the database. If the transaction failed, then the ROLLBACK statement is executed to reverse all completed steps in the transaction.

> ### NURSING ALERT
>
> The SQL statements used for transactions are dependent on the dialect of SQL used by the DBMS. Therefore, refer to the documentation provided by the DBMS vendor for SQL transaction statements for your DBMS.

This example shows a transaction that used to document the date and time of wound treatment in the patient medical record table and billing for the treatment in the patient bill table. You will notice NOW() is used in this transaction. NOW() is a function that returns the current date and time from the clock on the sever that is running the DBMS. The DBMS replaces NOW() with the current date and time.

```
START TRANSACTION
UPDATE PatientMRTB
    SET WoundTreatment = NOW()
    WHERE PatientMRN = "1234";
```

UPDATE PatientBillTB
   SET Treatment = "Wound", Charge = $540
   WHERE PatientMRN = "1234";

If processing is completed error free, then the COMMIT statement is executed.

COMMIT

If an error occurred during processing, then the ROLLBACK statement is executed.

   ROLLBACK

10. SQL Security

Restricting access to information in a database is the primary method of securing the information from threats. The most common way to restrict access is by using the **GRANT statement**. The GRANT statement enables you to give all access or specific access to a table. Access is called a right. Rights are:

- SELECT
- INSERT
- DELETE
- UPDATE

You give access by creating a **GRANT statement**. The GRANT statement requires the name of the right being granted, the name of the table, and the user ID who is being granted the right. In this example, we are giving the right to SELECT and INSERT on the PatientTB to BG1234, which is a user ID.

   GRANT SELECT, INSERT
      ON PatientTB
      TO BG1234;

Access can be removed by using the REVOKE statement. The REVOKE statement is structured nearly identical to the GRANT statement except REVOKE is used in place of GRANT as shown here.

   REVOKE SELECT, INSERT
      ON PatientTB
      TO BG1234;

Access can also be granted to selected columns. For example, a user can be restricted to retrieving only the patient's name and not the patient address. Access is granted by specifying column names within parentheses as shown here.

```
GRANT SELECT (PatientFirstName, PatientMiddleName,
PatientLastName)
   ON PatientTB
   TO BG1234;
```

Views

Another way to restrict access to information in the table is by creating a **view**. A view is a virtual table whose contents are defined by a query. To the database user, the view appears just like a real table and can be used like any table. A view is created using the CREATE VIEW statement. The CREATE VIEW statement specifies a name for the view and uses the AS clause to define a query that creates the view.

There are two types of views. These are:

- Horizontal view: A horizontal view contains all columns from a table and selected rows from the table.

- Vertical view: A vertical view contains selected columns from a table and all rows from the table.

The following example shows a horizontal view that displays rows from the PatientTB that contains MD1234 as the PractitionerID.

```
CREATE VIEW DrSmithPatients AS
   SELECT *
     FROM PatientTB
     WHERE PractitionerID = MD1234;
```

In the next example, we create a view called PatientName that contains the patient medical record number and patient name from the patient table. This is an example of a vertical view.

```
CREATE VIEW PatientName AS
   SELECT PatientMRN, PatientFirstName, PatientMiddleName,
   PatientLastName
     FROM PatientTB;
```

NURSING ALERT

Views are frequently used to limit access to clinical systems analyst, and MIS developers have to enter information in the database. A view can be created from a join (see Join), enabling the view to have all or some columns from both tables.

A view can be removed by using the DROP VIEW statement as shown here.

DROP VIEW PatientName;

11. Stored Procedures

When a request is made to a DBMS, the query is sent to the DBMS. For many clinical systems, this means that the query leaves the computer that sends the query and travels over a computer network to the database server that is running the DBMS and houses the database. For frequently used, large queries, the time to transmit the query is appreciable and may affect the response time. That is, response time is the time for the DBMS to process the query and reply to the query.

A more effect design is to store the query on the DBMS and call the query each time there is a need to execute the query. This is called a **stored procedure**. A stored procedure is a query that is given a name and is saved to the database. The name of the query is used in another query asking the DBMS to run the stored procedure.

A stored procedure is created by using the CREATE PROC statement as shown in this next example. The name of the stored procedure is PatientBillAlert. The AS clause is used to identify the query. You'll notice that this query is one created earlier in this chapter to return the patient medical record number for patients whose net amount is above the average net amount. Notice that the BEGIN and END clause is used to identify the beginning of and end of the stored procedure.

```
CREATE PROC PatientBillAlert AS
BEGIN
SELECT PatientMRN
   FROM PatientBillTB
   WHERE NetAmount > AVG(NetAmount)
END;
```

A stored procedure is called within another query by using the EXECUTE statement followed by the name of the stored procedure as shown here. Notice that the name of store procedure is followed by parenthesis.

```
EXECUTE PatientBillAlert ();
```

NURSING ALERT

A stored procedure can call another stored procedure by using the EXECUTE statement within the stored procedure.

Passing Values

Sometimes a stored procedure may require additional information that is only known when the stored procedure is called. Let's say that you want to display a list of patients for a particular practitioner. The practitioner's ID is not known until the stored procedure is called. We can address this problem by passing the stored procedure the practitioner's ID when the stored procedure is called. This is referred to as passing a value.

To pass a value to a procedure, we need to define a place holder for the value, which is commonly called a variable. A variable requires an at sign (@) followed by a name that we give the variable. This is shown in the next stored procedure. The variable is then used within the stored procedure in place of the actual value that will be passed to the stored procedure.

The query in this example is also one used previously in this chapter. The variable @PractitionerID is used as the place holder for the practitioner's ID, which will be passed to the stored procedure. Notice that we defined the variable immediately after the name of the stored procedure. The variable must be defined with a data type. You use the same data type as the data type of the corresponding column. In this example, PractitionerID is the column name that we defined previously in this chapter (see Create a Table).

```
CREATE PROC DisplayMDPatients
  @PractitionerID INTEGER
  AS
  BEGIN
    SELECT PatientMRN, PatientFirstName, PatientLastName, MD.
    PractitionerID, PractitionerFirstName, PractitionerLastName
      FROM PatientTB PT, PractitionerTB MD
      WHERE PT.PractitionerID = @PractitionerID;
  END
```

Call the stored procedure from within another query by using the EXECUTE statement followed by the name of the stored procedure and the value that you want to pass to the stored procedure. The value must be within parentheses as shown here where 12345 is the practitioner's ID.

```
EXECUTE PatientBillAlert (12345);
```
Drop A Stored Procedure

A stored procedure can be removed by using the DROP PROCEDURE statement followed by the name of the stored procedure as shown here:

```
DROP PROCEDURE DisplayMDPatients;
```

Triggers

A **trigger** is a stored procedure that is automatically called when an event occurs. Events are INSERT, DELETE, or UPDATE. When the DBMS detects an event, the DBMS executes the trigger without having been told to do so by a query.

A trigger is created by using the CREATE TRIGGER statement. The CREATE TRIGGER statement requires that you give the trigger a name that is followed by the ON clause. The ON clause specifies the name of the table that is involved in the event, that is, the table where the INSERT, DELETE, or UPDATE occurs. The AS clause is used to define the query that is to be executed when the event occurs.

In the following example, we insert a new row into the patient bill table whenever a new row is inserted into the patient table. The trigger is called InsertPatientBill. Notice that we set the net amount and gross amount to zero.

```
CREATE TRIGGER InsertPatientBill
   ON PatientTB
   FOR INSERT
   AS
     BEGIN
       INSERT INTO PatientBillTB
         VALUES  (INSERTED.PatientMRN, 0, 0);
       END
```

CASE STUDY

CASE 1

The executive nurse is reviewing the results of your needs analysis that identifies what the healthcare facility will require to implement an electronic medical record system. She noticed that you indicated a new position for a database administrator with the requirement that the database administrator be proficient in writing SQL. The executive nurse is concerned about increasing headcount that is not directly related to patient care. She asks you the following questions. What are your best responses?

QUESTION 1. Why do we need a database administrator?
ANSWER: A database administrator is a technologist who has expertise in installing, updating, and maintaining databases that are used by clinical applications such as the electronic medical records system. It is the database administrator's responsibility to ensure that the database is available 24/7. Furthermore, the database administrator will be proactive to avoid or mitigate risks that are inherent in a clinical database application.

QUESTION 2. Why must the database administer be skilled in SQL?
ANSWER: In addition to using SQL to interact with the database, the database administrator will use SQL to generate customized clinical reports that are not available from the electronic medical records application. The database administrator can bypass the electronic medical records application and access the database directly. The nurse informatics specialist may be able to write reports if the nurse informatics specialists is proficient in SQL and has access to the database.

QUESTION 3. Will accessing the database directly using SQL void our contract with the vendor of the electronic medical records application?
ANSWER: Depending on the vendor selection, the healthcare facility may have limited rights to access the database directly. The limitation is typically to retrieve information stored in the database. That is, the database administrator will not be permitted to bypass the electronic medical records application to enter information or change existing information in the database. Some vendors do not permit any access to the database.

QUESTION 4. Why won't the vendor prevent us from accessing the database directly for any reason?
ANSWER: The vendor warrants that the clinical information acquired, processed, and stored by the electronic medical records application is accurate and compliant with regulatory authority. To offer the warranty, the vendor must have full control over the application and the database. Interacting directly with the database that violates the vendor contract voids the warranty, and therefore the vendor is no longer responsible for the accuracy of the information stored in the database or that the data is in compliance with regulatory requirements.

FINAL CHECK-UP

1. **What is SQL?**
   A. SQL is a type of programming language designed to build database applications.
   B. SQL is a type of programming language specifically designed to interact with DBMS to retrieve and manipulate information in the clinical database.
   C. SQL is a DBMS that stores and manipulates clinical data.
   D. SQL is a type of database specifically designed to retrieve and manipulate clinical information.

2. **Where are queries written?**
   A. Queries are embedded into programs or entered into an SQL console.
   B. Queries are embedded into programs.
   C. Queries are entered into an SQL console.
   D. Queries are written by the clinical staff to retrieve information from the database.

3. **Why is it important to use a naming convention?**
   A. A naming convention standardizes how names of columns are written, making the names easy for the DBMS to read and identify the kind of information stored in the column.
   B. A naming convention standardizes how names of columns are written, making the names easy for the person writing or reading the query to read and identify the kind of information stored in the column.
   C. A naming convention standardizes how names of columns are written, making the names easy to read and identify the kind of information stored in the column.
   D. Naming conventions are required by the DBMS.

4. **How do you specify search criteria in a query?**
   A. Use the WHERE clause.
   B. Use the SELECT clause.
   C. Use the FROM clause.
   D. Use the VALUES clause.

5. **How is data in a table summarized in a query?**
   A. Column functions.
   B. Use the WHERE clause.
   C. Use the FROM clause.
   D. Use the VALUES clause.

6. **How are two tables combined using a query?**

   A. Using a dataflow diagram

   B. Using naming conventions

   C. Using a join

   D. Using the ORDER BY statement

7. **What is the purpose of the TRANSACTION statement?**

   A. A TRANSACTION statement defines a transaction application.

   B. A TRANSACTION statement creates a transaction table.

   C. A TRANSACTION statement creates a transaction database.

   D. The TRANSACTION statement defines a group of SQL statements that form a transaction.

8. **What is a stored procedure?**

   A. A stored procedure is a frequently used query that is stored within a clinical database application.

   B. A stored procedure is a query that resides on the DBMS and can be executed by calling the name of the stored procedure in an SQL statement.

   C. A stored procedure is a frequently used query.

   D. A stored procedure is a query that resides on the DBMS.

9. **What is the benefit of using stored procedures?**

   A. A stored procedure reduces the transmission time necessary to execute a query.

   B. A stored procedure is a requirement of all clinical information systems.

   C. Stored procedures are required by HIPPA law to protect access to patient information.

   D. A stored procedure is a way a clinical application complies with HIPPA.

10. **What clause is used in a query to remove duplicate values being returned by the DBMS?**

    A. GROUP BY clause

    B. Column functions

    C. Distinct clause

    D. HAVING clause

CORRECT ANSWERS AND RATIONALES

1. B. SQL is a type of programming language specifically designed to interact with DBMS to retrieve and manipulate information in the clinical database.
2. A. Queries are embedded into programs or entered into an SQL console.
3. B. A naming convention standardizes how names of columns are written, making the names easy for the person writing or reading the query to read and identify the kind of information stored in the column.
4. A. Use the WHERE clause.
5. A. Column functions.
6. C. Using a join.
7. D. The TRANSACTION statement defines a group of SQL statements that form a transaction.
8. B. A stored procedure is a query that resides on the DBMS and can be executed by calling the name of the stored procedure in an SQL statement.
9. A. A stored procedure reduces transmission time necessary to execute a query.
10. C. Distinct clause.

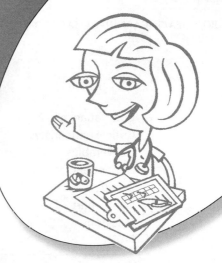

chapter 5

Clinical Project Management

LEARNING OBJECTIVES

1. Introduction to project management
2. Work breakdown structure and tasks
3. Resources
4. Costs
5. Management tools
6. Change management
7. Risk management
8. Postdevelopment
9. Agile project management

KEY TERMS

Cost variance
Critical path analysis
Deliverables
Dependencies
Duration
Gantt chart
Milestones
Project

Project charter
Project life cycle
Project phase
Resource allocation
Scope statement
Tasks
Work breakdown structure
Work plan

1. Introduction to Project Management

A **project** is a temporary set of activities that delivers a unique outcome. A project is temporary, requires resources, is unique, and has a project sponsor who has requested that the project be undertaken. Project management is applying project management skills and tools to transform an idea into reality. Project management skills and tools include a methodology to manage the transformation. The methodology is a set of proven techniques that increases success and minimizes risk during the transformation.

In this chapter, you will learn about tools used by project manager to apply a methodology that turns an idea into reality. Those tools include:

- **Project charter**: A project charter specifies what the project manager is to deliver and the terms under which the project manager will manage the project.

- **Scope statement**: A scope statement is a brief expression of what will be delivered.

- **Work plan**: The work plan is a detailed description and organization of **tasks** and resource that are necessary to complete the project.

- **Gantt chart**: A Gantt chart is a visual depiction of the work plan.

- **Critical path analysis**: The critical path analysis determines tasks that will affect the **duration** of the project. That is, a change in the duration of tasks that fall on the critical path affects the duration of the project.

- Cost estimates: A cost estimate is the project manager's projected cost of the project.

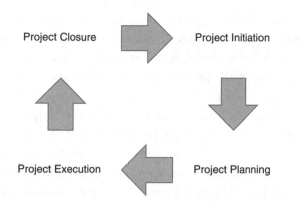

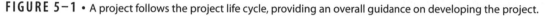

FIGURE 5−1 • A project follows the project life cycle, providing an overall guidance on developing the project.

The Project Life Cycle

Every project follows a predictable course referred to as the **project life cycle** (Figure 5–1). The project life cycle consists of four stages. The first is the project initiation stage during which an idea for a project is fully developed and justified. Next is the project planning stage. It is here when the project manager takes the idea and develops a plan to turn the idea into a reality. The project planning stage is followed by the project execution stage, which is when the project is built based on the project manager's plans. The final stage is the project closure stage. This is when the project is implemented.

Project Initiation

During the project initiation stage, the project sponsor identifies the clinical need for the project and develops a clinical case for launching the project. The clinical case typically is based on new regulatory requirements, patient safety, or a more efficient and effective means of providing quality care to patients.

In addition to making the clinical case, the project sponsor identifies constraints of the project. A constraint is usually time, money, availability of resources, and limitations posed by the clinical environment. The project sponsor also identifies assumptions that provide the foundation for determining that the project will be beneficial to the healthcare facility. For example, the project sponsor may want wireless computers on wheels (COWs) based on the anticipation of increased census due to the opening of a specialty unit. The list of assumptions is reviewed throughout the course of development to assess if assumptions are valid. A change in an assumption might weaken the clinical case for the project and may cause the cancellation of the project.

The project sponsor writes a scope statement. A scope statement briefly describes the purpose of the project and is used throughout the project's development to keep stakeholders and the project team focused on the project's goal.

The project initiation stage concludes when the project sponsor and the project manager develop a charter for the project. Think of a charter as a contract between the project sponsor and the project manager. The project charter lists the project sponsor's expectations, the scope statement, limitations and constraints within which the project is to be developed, and a timeline for delivering the project.

Project Planning

The project planning stage is the time when the project manager takes over the project and translates the project sponsor's idea into reality. Planning begins with **work breakdown structure** (WBS) (see Work Breakdown Structure and Tasks). The WBS is a process whereby the project manager looks at the expected deliverable (the whole) and then breaks down the expected deliverable into a work package (a part of the whole). The project manager then determines tasks needed to create the work package.

Let's say that the project sponsor wants to implement an electronic medical record administration record (eMAR). The whole is the eMAR application. A work group might be administration of medication using the eMAR. That is, how does a nurse administer medication using the eMAR?

The project manager then develops a plan for building each work package. The plan details all tasks—and when those tasks are to be performed—that must be accomplished to complete the work package. The plan also identifies and assigns resourses to each task. A resource is a person(s) who performs the tasks and things that the person needs to perform the task. After resources are assigned to a task, the project manager calculates the cost of performing the task. The project manager estimates the cost of the project by adding together the cost for each task. The project manager also considers the timeline and other constraints and limitations specified in the charter when developing the plan.

Project Execution

The project execution stage is when the project team comes together to make the project sponsor's idea a reality by following the project plan developed by the project manager. It is during this period when the project manager fine tunes the project plan to adjust for changes that might occur during the course of development. The project manager's and the project team's focus is on monitoring and controlling all elements that develop to ensure that the project remains within the scope of the project, on schedule, and on budget.

Project Closure

The project closure stage begins after the project is fully developed and has passed all tests. The next step is for the project sponsor and stakeholders to verify that the product delivered by the project team is acceptable. This is done by performing a user acceptance test. After it is accepted, the project manager develops a plan to migrate from the existing system to the new system. Migration includes training staff, converting data, and doing everything necessary to make the system useable by the stakeholders.

After the system is live, the project manager and project team review the project and learns what went right and what could have gone better. These are called lessons learned. The project plan and other documents used on the project are archived, and the project team disbands.

2. Work Breakdown Structure and Tasks

Imagine that you are the project manager who has been given the task to develop an eMAR. In essence, the project sponsor simply says, "Build me an eMAR." Your job is to make this idea a reality. The question that you need to answer for yourself is, "Where do we begin?"

The answer is to begin with the work breakdown structure (WBS). All project planning begins with the WBS. A WBS begins with the end objective and successively subdivides the end objective into manageable components. The end component is referred to as a work package.

A work package is the lowest level of the work breakdown structure and consists of a group of tasks. It is the work package level where all the work is performed. Think of a work package as a piece of the whole thing. When one work package is completed, then one piece of the whole is completed. The entire project is completed when all work packages are completed.

The concept of a WBS is easy to understand, but implementing a WBS can be challenging because it is difficult to know when to stop breaking down the work. The best approach is to use the common-sense rule. That is, if it makes sense, then break down the work further. If the activity produces a deliverable package of work that is measurable, then do not break down the work further.

Figure 5–2 provides a relatively brief WBS of an eMAR.

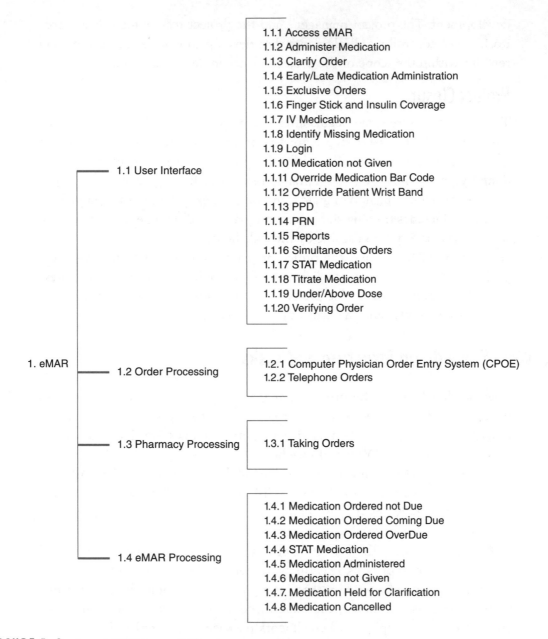

FIGURE 5-2 • A partial WBS for an eMAR system.

Project Phase, Milestones, and Deliverables

A project can be divided into phases. A **project phase** is delivering a discrete product such as implementing an eMAR to acute units of a healthcare facility. A second phase might be to implement the eMAR to the clinic. Another phase may be to implement the eMAR to the surgical units. Each phase has a start and finish date and its own project plan, schedule, and budget. The project team moves on to the next phase of the project after a phase is completed.

Progress toward the end of the project is measured in **milestones** and **deliverables**. A milestone is an event that identifies a significant accomplishment in developing the project. For example, creating a barcode-based inventory of all medication packages is a milestone as is training all nurses to use the eMAR.

A deliverable is the result of performing a task. For example, Nexium was added to the barcode-based inventory, and five nurses in the cardiac care unit were trained to use eMAR. These are deliverables. However, these are not milestones because they do not show significant progress toward the end of the project.

> **NURSING ALERT**
>
> A milestone is a measurement of significant progress. A deliverable is the result of a task.

Task and Subtask

A work group is divided into tasks. A task is an action that has a beginning and an end that produces a result. A task can be divided into one or more subtasks. A subtask is an action that has a beginning and an end and produces a result that is used as an action of another task.

For example, a task might be to design the data entry screen of the eMAR. Subtasks are to meet with nurses, physicians, nurse practitioners, and pharmacists and gather input regarding their requirements for the screen.

A task can be related to other tasks. For example, one task may not be able to start until another task finishes. This is called task relationships. The project manager must identify tasks, subtasks, and task relationships for every work package. Here are commonly used task relationships:

- Finish-to-start: You cannot start designing the entry screen before gathering the requirements.
- Start-to-start: Start designing the entry screen and start designing the data validation process.

- Finish-to-finish: Finish designing the entry screen and finish designing the data validation process.

- Start-to-finish: Gathering requirements determines the finish date of when the design of the entry screen is completed.

Sequencing Task

After task relationships are identified, the project manager then determines the sequencing of task, that is, which tasks are performed first, second, and so on and what tasks can be performed concurrently. Sequencing is based on **dependencies** of tasks. A dependency exists when another task cannot start or cannot finish until another task finishes.

Project managers review tasks and attributes, project scope statement, and milestones to determine the dependencies among activities. The project manager then answers these questions:

- Does a task need to be finished before another one can start?

- Can several tasks be done concurrently?

- Can some tasks overlap?

NURSING ALERT

Task sequencing impacts the project schedule.

Duration

Duration is the length of time resources work on a task plus elapsed time. For example, a task might take 1 week to complete, but the duration may be 2 weeks because of resource availability. Duration is estimated by a standard measurement of time. The standard has to be determined at the beginning of a project. For example, duration can be measured in days; however, a day must be defined such as an 8-hour day or a 7.5-hour day. This becomes important, especially if resources are expensed by the hour. Measuring duration in workdays or work hours is called effort.

The project manager must determine the duration for all tasks. You can imagine this is challenging because the project manager probably has never performed any of those tasks. Here are common techniques used to estimate duration—and its primary disadvantage:

- Prior experience (analogous) estimating: No two projects are alike.

- Historic statistical relationships (parametric) estimating: History may not repeat itself.

- Expert judgment (subject matter expert): The expert may not have the time or inclination to gather all the facts to produce a realistic estimate. The expert may not be an expert and may have no vested interest in the estimate—nothing to lose if the estimate is wrong.
- Bottom-up (decomposition) estimate: Analysis of the details of all tasks and subtask takes time.

There is no perfect method of estimating duration. There are too many variables that influence the duration. A good approach is to ask the person, who is going to perform the task, how much time is necessary to perform the task. This is different than asking an expert because the person is committed to completing the task. That is, the person has something to lose if the task is behind schedule.

When arriving at an estimate, make sure that you record any assumptions made by the person giving the estimate such as hours in a day, availability of staff, and availability of resources. Monitor the underlying assumptions during the project. Any change in the underlying assumption might affect the actual duration of the task.

Also determine if the task is effort driven (variable duration) or duration driven (fixed duration). Variable duration means that you can add more resources to the task to reduce the duration. Fixed duration means that adding more resources to the task will not reduce the duration.

Schedule Development

The project manager can develop a schedule for the project after the tasks and subtasks are identified, the duration is established, and the relationships among tasks are defined. The schedule will specify when each task begins and ends and collectively when the project begins and ends. The project manager and the project team easily know what activity is occurring at any moment during the project. In addition, the project manager can estimate the impact of task change on the entire project.

The critical path is also determined after the schedule is developed. The critical path consists of tasks that impact the delivery of the project. Increasing the duration of a task that is on the critical path extends the delivery of the project. Shortening the duration of a task that is on the critical path may shorten the delivery of the project. Tasks tend to fall on and off the critical path depending on the schedule. For example, a shortened task that is on the critical path may cause the task to fall off the critical path and another task to take its place on the critical path.

Tasks and subtasks are typically entered into project management software that automatically generates an image of the schedule in the form of a Gantt

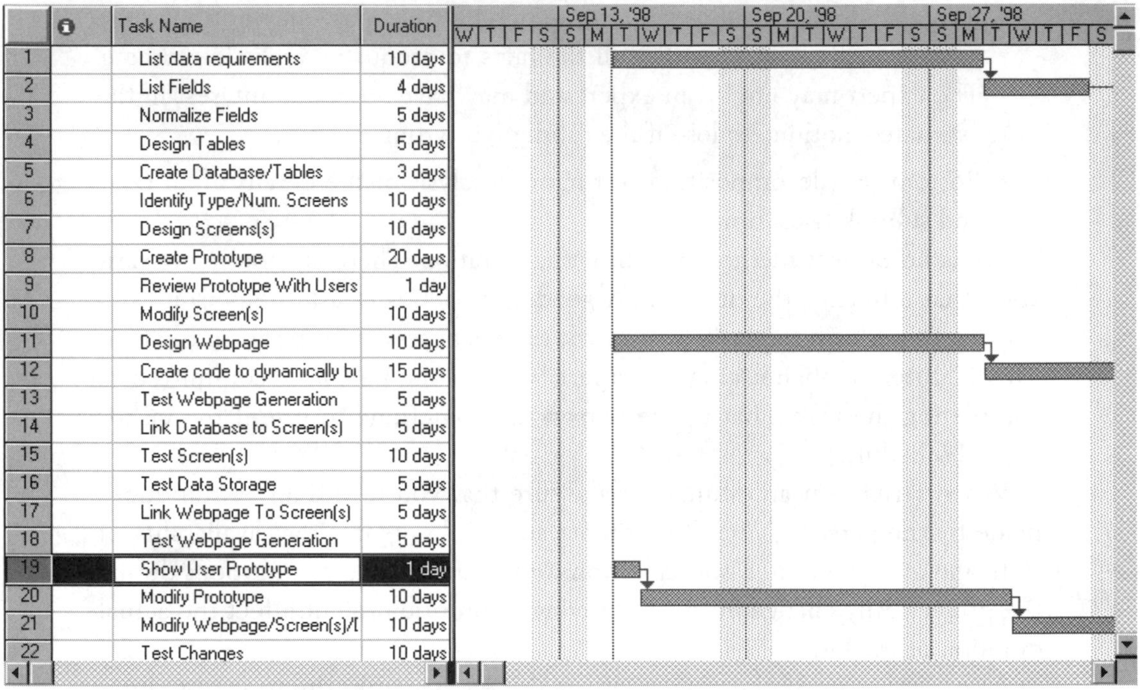

3

FIGURE 5–3 • A Gantt chart depicts tasks, duration, and dependencies on a calendar that makes viewing the project easy.

chart (Figure 5–3). A Gantt chart lists tasks and subtasks and plots durations as bars across a calendar. Dependencies among tasks are shown as a line that connects the bars of the tasks. Project management software also calculates the impact of changes to tasks and revises the Gantt chart to reflect the changes.

> **NURSING ALERT**
> Microsoft Project is a commonly used project management software.

3. Resources

A resource is a thing or person required to complete a task or subtask. The project manager must identify all resources for each task. This can become challenging because some of the most obvious resources are overlooked.

Let's say that a task is to develop specifications for the proposed eMAR system. Intuitively, you rightfully assume that you require a clinical systems analyst as a resource to perform the task. Ask yourself, what does the clinical systems analyst require to perform the task? You might say a computer, a telephone, paper, a pen, and maybe a printer. These, too, are correct. Other resources are also needed such as office space, a desk, chair, electricity, heat, air conditioning, lights, a parking space, access to the facility, and other resources that are typically assumed to be available but may not be available.

A good way to assess resources for a task is to assume no resource exists and that you must supply everything needed to perform a task. Begin with a person who will perform the task such as a clinical systems analyst. Picture the person standing in the doorway of the person's home ready to go to your healthcare facility. List everything the person needs to do her job. Mentally follow the person through the steps to do her work.

For example, the person drives from home to the facility and needs to park her car. The person needs identification to enter the healthcare facility. The person needs to go somewhere after she has access to the facility (i.e., office space). By following the person's path, the project manager is able to list all resources needed to perform the task.

Acquire Resources

The next step is to focus on tasks required to acquire resources. Let's begin by looking at tasks required to acquire a clinical systems analyst. Here is a list of tasks:

- Write a job description.
- Set a salary range based on the healthcare facility's salary scale.
- Write the justification for the position.
- Submit a form for new headcount for approval.
- Submit a request for a new employee to human resources.
- Human resources posts the job position in-house for 10 days.
- Human resources reviews in-house applicants.
- Human resources posts the job position for nonemployees.
- Human resources reviews resumes.
- Human resources gives the project manager five qualified candidates.
- Human resources interviews candidates.
- The project manager interviews candidates.
- The project manager informs human resources to hire one candidate.
- Human resources sends the candidate an offer and terms of employment.

- Human resources negotiates the terms of employment with the candidate.
- The candidate accepts the offer.
- A start date is set.

The project manager needs to determine the duration for each task and resources needed to perform each task. For example, collectively, the duration may be 3 months before the clinical systems analyst start date arrives. These tasks—and duration—become part of the project plan.

Other factors must be considered in this example. The new employee is unlikely to be productive for several weeks as she settles into a new job and work environment. Think of this as the honeymoon period during which the new hire and the project manager get to know each other. The duration of the honeymoon period must be considered in the schedule because it impacts the duration of the task assigned to the new hire.

And what happens if the new hire is unable to perform some or the entire task? The project manager must decide if the new hire will remain on the project team. If the new hire is able to perform some of the task, then the project manager may have to redefine the task or identify another resource to work with the new hire on the task—and then acquire that resource. If the new hire is unable to perform the task, then the project manager must begin the hiring process again. All of this impacts the project schedule.

Do not underestimate the time necessary to acquire a resource. From the time the project manager recognizes a need for a clinical systems analyst to the time when the clinical systems analyst is productively working on the task can be 4 or 5 months. Acquiring office space could take 3 to 6 months depending on availability. Acquiring a resource can appreciably extend the duration of the project.

Tasks to acquire a resource should be included in the project schedule and be depicted in the Gantt chart. All tasks to acquire a resource should have the same end date. The end date is the beginning date of tasks needed to complete the project. That is, all tasks to acquire a resource should be completed when the task to be performed by the resource begins.

The project manager can calculate when to begin the task of acquiring a resource by referring to the end date (i.e., when the resource needs to be on board and productive) and the duration of acquiring the resource. For example, the project manager knows that she must begin the hiring process for a clinical systems analyst 4 months before beginning the task to develop specifications for the proposed eMAR system.

			Resource Name	Initials	Group	Max. Units	Std. Rate	Ovt. Rate	Cost/Use	Accrue At	Base Cale
	1	◇	Business Analyst	B		100%	$0.00/hr	$0.00/hr	$0.00	Prorated	Standard
	2	◇	System Analyst	S		100%	$0.00/hr	$0.00/hr	$0.00	Prorated	Standard
	3	◇	User Manager	U		100%	$0.00/hr	$0.00/hr	$0.00	Prorated	Standard
	4	◇	Day-To-Day User	D		100%	$0.00/hr	$0.00/hr	$0.00	Prorated	Standard
	5	◇	DBA	D		100%	$0.00/hr	$0.00/hr	$0.00	Prorated	Standard
	6	◇	Programmer 1 scrn	P		100%	$0.00/hr	$0.00/hr	$0.00	Prorated	Standard
	7	◇	Programmer 2 web	P		100%	$0.00/hr	$0.00/hr	$0.00	Prorated	Standard

Task Usage

Tracking Gantt

Resource Graph

FIGURE 5–4 • A resource list contains all resources available to work on tasks along with each resource's cost and availability.

Not all resources are needed the first day of a project. Likewise, some resources are nice to have but are not required. Therefore, the project manager must prioritize when resources must be acquired and then focus on acquiring resources based on the priority list. For example, a clinical systems analyst may be able to share office space until permanent office space becomes available.

Resource List

The project manager needs to create a list of resources commonly referred to as a resource list after resources are acquired and available to work (Figure 5–4). The resource list contains a resource by title, the availability of the resource to the project, and the cost of the resource. Each title should be unique. For example, there might be more than one clinical systems analyst; therefore, the title should be clinical systems analyst 1, clinical systems analyst 2, and so on.

Some resources may not be available 100% of the time to the project. A resource that is in high demand may be shared among several projects and be available a portion of the resource's time to a particular project. For example, a resource may be available 50% of the resource time to the project. This is noted in the resource list.

The cost of the resource is the per unit amount that is charged to the project for use of the resource. In some organizations, a clinical systems analyst is charged to the project an hourly amount that represents salary and benefits. In other organizations, a clinical systems analyst is charged as a daily amount. The cost is listed in the resource list and is used as a multiplier for the amount of time spent on the task to determine the cost of the task. This calculation is performed by the project management software.

NURSING ALERT

Do not use a person's name in the resource list. Always use a title. More than one person can fill the role during the life cycle of the project. The project manager assigns a person to the title.

Resource Allocation

Resource allocation is the process of assigning resources to tasks. Only resources that appear on the resource list can be allocated to a task. These are resources that have been identified and acquired to work on the project. Resources are assigned to each task by using features in the project management software. The Gantt chart displays abbreviations for resources alongside the task depending on the project management software in use.

After allocating resources, the project manager assesses the allocation of resources using the allocation chart. The allocation chart depicts the percentage of the resource's available time that is allocated for each day of the project. The available time (see Resource List) is 100% of time in the allocation chart. For example, a resource available half a day will appear 100% allocated if the resource is assigned to a task that requires 4 hours' work for that day assuming a workday is 8 hours long.

An allocation over 100% indicates that the resource is asked to perform more than a day's work in a day. Overallocation is a common occurrence when the project manager initially allocates resources because the project manager is focused on tasks rather than a resource's allocation.

The project manager must revisit the need of resources and the allocation of resources if a resource is overallocated. For example, the project manager may consider rearranging tasks so that tasks can be performed in sequence rather than consecutively enabling the resource to complete the first task before working on the next task. Alternatively, the project manager may assign a different resource to the task.

The goal is to allocate all resources at 100%. Sometimes slight overallocation is acceptable. For example, a resource allocated at 150% for 1 day may be asked to work overtime (Figure 5–5). One hundred percent is 8 hours, and an additional 4 hours of overtime (50%) will have the resource work a 12-hour work day. Overtime is an exception and not the rule. Productivity decreases as overtime increases.

After resources are properly allocated, the project manager can use the project management software to produce a work schedule for each

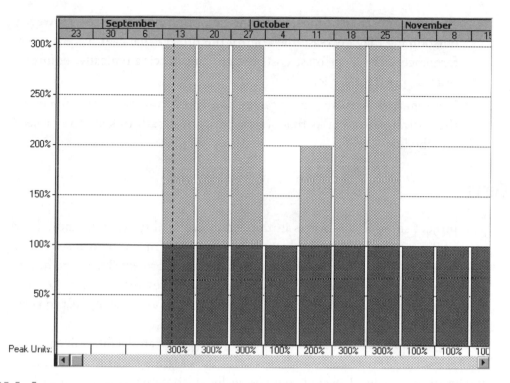

FIGURE 5–5 · A resource that is overallocated is displayed in grey. Assignments need to be reallocated to avoid over-allocating the resource.

resource that clearly depicts what the resource is scheduled to do and when to do it.

Resource Usage

There are techniques a project manager can use to manage the usage of resources. These are:

- Use a less expensive resource: This may lower the cost of performing a task; however, the project manager must assess the impact on the quality of work and if the resource may be less productive, leading to an increased duration of the task.

- Use a more expensive resource: This may increase the cost of the task; however, productivity may increase, and the duration of the task may decrease.

- Overallocate: A resource that works overtime may decrease the duration of a task; however, the cost of the task may increase.

- Outsource: Assigning a task or a group of tasks to another organization may decrease overallocation of existing resources and provide an alternative to the time-consuming task of hiring a resource. However, outsourcing may decrease the control the project manager has over performance and may increase costs because outsourcing typically requires a priming price for service.

- Reassign resources: Resources can be reassigned from tasks that are not on the critical path to tasks that are on the critical path to keep the project on schedule.

4. Costs

The project sponsor and others in the healthcare facility want to know how much a project will cost, and they turn to the project manager to answer that question. Generally, there are two types of cost for a project. These are development cost and ongoing cost. Development cost represents the cost of everything to create and implement the system. Ongoing cost represents cost to keep the system running.

Let's take the eMAR system as an example. Healthcare facilities license the eMAR system from a vendor and then tailor the eMAR system to the needs of the healthcare facility. Development cost includes a one-time cost for the eMAR software and installation and the cost of the clinical systems analyst to use software tools provided by the vendor to tailor the eMAR system to the needs of the healthcare facility. Also included is one-time training cost of the staff. Ongoing cost includes the annual software license for the product, upgrades to the software, operation of the computers running the eMAR and the network used to distribute eMAR data, and management information systems (MIS) staff to maintain the eMAR software and hardware. Also included is ongoing training of new staff.

Development cost is determined by estimating the work and material involved in completing tasks. Work is the time a resource worked on the task (e.g., clinical systems analyst) and material is the cost of resources used to perform the task (e.g., travel). Most of the cost is calculated by the project management software if the project manager included cost factors for each resource on the resource list. Other costs not available to the project management software must be calculated manually.

Cost Variance

The project manager estimates the cost of the entire project and incurs actual cost during the development process. The difference between estimate and actual cost is called a **cost variance**. The goal is to have zero cost variance.

However, there will always be a cost variance because not all factors are known when the costs are estimated, and assumptions that are the basis for the estimate may change during the course of development.

Cost variance is measured using a cost performance index (CPI) and is calculated using the following formula: CPI = Estimated cost/Actual cost. A perfect CPI is 1. Less than 1 means that the actual cost is higher than the estimated cost. More than 1 means that the actual cost is lower than the estimated cost. Project managers use the CPI through the development process to gauge cost.

The finance department of some healthcare facilities believes that a cost variance of +/− 10% of the estimate is acceptable. A greater cost variance requires the project manager to justify the difference. That is, the project manager has to review the estimate to determine why the estimate was off target.

> ### NURSING ALERT
>
> Whenever there is a change in the scope of a project, the project manager develops another cost estimate that includes the change. Therefore, changes in the scope of the project have no impact on a cost variance.

Cost Estimating Techniques

Project managers use one of two techniques to estimate the cost of a project. These are a top-down estimate and a bottom-up estimate. A top-down estimate is based on a gross comparison of the project with another similar project that has already been implemented and whose actual cost is known. The benefits of a top-down estimate are that the estimate can be arrived at quickly, and the estimate isn't expensive to produce. The drawback is that no two projects are exactly the same, and therefore the estimate is less accurate than the bottom-up estimate technique.

The bottom-up estimate technique requires the project manager to identify tasks, duration of tasks, and resources for the project first and then summarize the estimated cost of each task. The benefit of the bottom-up estimate is accuracy because the cost analysis is based on the project, not a different project. The drawback is that the bottom-up estimate technique is timely and therefore costly to produce.

Some project managers use both methods for estimating a project. The top-down estimate is used to produce a magnitude estimate occasionally called a "ballpark" estimate. A magnitude estimate is used by a project sponsor to determine if a project is economically feasible. This is similar in concept to what you might use when buying a car and asking for a price range to determine if the price is within your budget. A project manager determines a top-down estimate by finding a recently implemented similar project and then roughly identifies differences in the proposed project from the implemented project that impact the cost. The estimate is adjusted for escalated costs since a similar project was implemented for contingencies and situations that may arise during the proposed project. The project manager also documents the rationale for the estimate.

If the project sponsor determines that the project is financially feasible and is likely to be approved, the project manager uses project specifications and the bottom-up estimate technique to fine tune the estimate. If the estimate is above the amount expected by the project sponsor, the project manager can then adjust the project plan at the task level to bring the estimated cost more in line with expectations.

5. Management Tools

Many elements used to organize a project become tools that the project manager uses to manage the project (see Introduction to Project Management). These are the scope statement, project charter, project plan, Gantt chart, schedule, and status reports.

The scope statement is a brief statement—a sentence or paragraph—that specifies the goal of the project. The project manager can use the scope statement as a reminder to the project team of the goal. Some project managers place the scope statement in every communication document such as in a header or at the end of the document. Likewise, the scope statement is on a banner or poster in meeting rooms.

The project charter is the contract between the project team and the project sponsor and lists the goals, constraints, and other terms within which the project is developed. The project manager uses the project charter as a working tool throughout the project and shares the project charter with the project team. The project manager and the project team refer to the project charter during all decision-making processes to ensure that the decision complies with the project charter.

The project plan is the step-by-step guide on how the project sponsor's idea is transformed into reality. The project plan is referenced before any decision is made about the project. A key element of the project plan is the critical path (Figure 5–6). The critical path contains tasks whose change in duration changes the duration of the project. Many project managers consult the critical path when making personnel decisions such as granting time off from work.

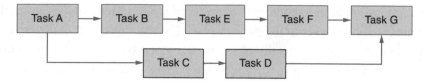

FIGURE 5–6 • The critical path identifies tasks whose change in duration affects the duration of the project.

The Gantt chart is a visual image of the project plan showing all tasks, duration, dependencies, and resource allocation. Some managers share the Gantt chart with the project team, enabling each team member to see his task relationship to all tasks of the project.

The project plan is the basis for the schedule. The schedule is a list of task assignments along with start and end dates for each project team member. Some project managers distribute the schedule to each member weekly or monthly.

Status reports are updates on how well the project is following the project plan. The project manager develops various status reports, each designed to meet the needs of a particular audience. There are different people interested in the project, and each has their own interest. At the beginning of the project, the project manager identifies people such as the project sponsor, stakeholders, and financial managers who require updates on the project. Next, the project manager asks each the type, format, frequency, and method of delivery of the information. Status reports are then assembled to meet those requirements.

> **NURSING ALERT**
>
> A project management tool such as Microsoft Project has reports that can be automatically generated by the software, which reduces the effort to produce status reports.

6. Change Management

Change management is a process that is initiated at the beginning of the project to deal with changes in the project scope after the project is approved. In the ideal world, project specifications and the scope of the project would not change after the project charter is defined and specifications agreed upon by the project sponsor, the stakeholders, and the project team. However, change is expected throughout the life of the project as system analysts, business analysts, and stakeholders take a close look at business processes and decide that processes can be performed more efficiently.

In many projects, enhancements are wanted when specifications are defined and squeezed into the existing project plan. That is, there is pressure to incorporate change without officially changing the scope of the project or changing the project plan, resulting in a project that is over budget and delayed. This is commonly referred to as scope creep.

The project manager and the project sponsor must recognize that everything is not known about a project when the project is launched, that important enhancements will likely be discovered during the course of development, and that these enhancements must be included in the project plan. Recognizing that the project scope and specifications will probably change, the project manager and the project sponsor should develop a structure to accommodate change, which is called a change management process.

The change management process is a structure within which enhancements to the project can be proposed at any time during the project development. Each proposed enhancement will be brought before a change management committee established by the project sponsor. The person making the proposal is called the owner of the enhancement and is required to present the advantages and disadvantages of incorporating the enhancement into the project plan. Furthermore, the enhancement owner with the assistance of the project manager will present the duration and cost of the enhancement.

The change management committee then determines if the enhancement is worth the impact to the deadline and cost of the project. The change management committee also decides if the enhancement will be part of the project. If so, the project manager revises the project plan, deliverables, milestones, and other aspects to incorporate the enhancement into the project plan. Likewise, the projected cost of the project is revised to reflect the enhancement.

The existing project plan and budget are replaced by the revised project plan and budget. Everyone involved in the project is told to disregard previously announced schedules, deadlines, and budgets. New schedules, deadlines, and budgets are then provided to everyone. These revisions contain the approved enhancement.

7. Risk Management

Every project has risk associated with it. There is a risk that funding will no longer be available and the project is terminated before completion. There is a risk that resources required for tasks on the critical path will not be available. And there are risks that underlying assumptions as the basis for the project plan are wrong.

Risks are inherent in every project, and there is no way to eliminate risk no matter how carefully you plan a project. However, you can take steps to reduce exposure to risk and develop contingency plans that can be implemented to mitigate problems if they occur by creating a risk management plan.

A risk management plan identifies fail points in a project. A fail point is a situation in which something can fail and therefore presents as a risk to the successful completion of the project. Identify fail points by carefully examining each facet of the project and assess the likelihood for success. That is, assess the probability that what you plan will be realized.

For example, a clinical analyst is needed to create process specifications for documenting an admission assessment in the patient's electronic medical record. The presumption is that the clinical analyst has the skillset to complete the task and will work 5 days a week for 6 consecutive weeks. There are two fail points in this scenario, that is, the clinical analyst has the necessary skillset and that the clinical analyst will work the expected amount of time. There is no guarantee that one or both of these fail points will fail.

A fail point typically falls into one of several categories of risk. These are:

- Inherent risk: Inherent risk is a natural risk that exists in any project. For example, key employees are unable to work because of illness.

- Business risk: Business risk is a risk associated with doing business. That is, the business falls under adverse market conditions.

- Detection risk: Detection risk is a risk that occurs because the clinical project manager or an advisor uses faulty procedures or bases a decision on unknowingly false information. For example, the duration for a task is set based on invalid historical data.

- Technological risk: Technological risk is the chance that a key system will fail such as the infrastructure being unable to handle the data load.

- Operational risk: Operational risk happens when the business logic is faulty, resulting in unexpected outcomes from the project.

- Residual risk: Residual risk is a risk that remains after the clinical project manager has mitigated other risks.

Risk Response

Each fail point must be assessed for the probability that the negative event will occur and the impact that occurrence has on the project. Based on this assessment, the clinical project manager decides how to respond to the risk. The response is based on the risk tolerance of clinical project manager and the organization concerning the impact the project has on the facility.

There are four common responses a clinical project manager can have for each fail point. These are:

- Accept: The clinical project manager acknowledges and ignores the risk. This is a common response for fail points that have a low probability of occurrence or have a large effort to mitigate or avoid. The decision is to take your chances rather than take a proactive stance to address the risk.

- Mitigate: A fail point that might have a relatively low chance of occurring, but has a major impact on the project if it does occur should not be ignored. Instead, a reasonable effort can be made to do something that lowers the probability that the fail point will fail. This is referred to as mitigation. Mitigation lowers the probability of occurrence by taking a proactive role in trying to prevent the occurrence.

- Transfer: A risk can be moved to another party, thereby limiting the risk to the clinical project manager. For example, the clinical project manager may decide to outsource a portion of the project. Risk associated with fail points associated with that portion of the project are transferred to the outsource firm. Of course, the risk still exists, and an occurrence that will impact the project is something that the clinical project manager must address.

- Avoid: The clinical project manager may decide that the fail point has a high probability of occurring and therefore an effort must be made to remove the fail point from the project. This is typically addressed by redesigning the project to avoid the fail point.

Risk Management Plan

A risk management plan is developed by the clinical project manager to either mitigate or transfer the risk. It consists of contingencies that can be implemented if a risk is realized. Some clinical project managers commonly refer to the risk management plan as "plan B and plan C" in case "plan A" fails.

The risk management plan should contain likely and unlikely scenarios that might occur and procedures that should be followed if they do occur. The objective is to devise solid fallback plans before a fail point event occurs. Events are clearly identified, and all actions are predefined. If an event occurs, the clinical project manager identifies the corresponding component in the risk management plan and executes the corresponding predefined actions.

The goal is to minimize the need to define contingencies when an event occurs. For example, a clinical project manager may have preliminary arrangements with an outsource firm to take over a key component of the project in case one or more members of the project team are unable to work on the project. When the clinical project manager realizes the staffing problem, the outsource firm is called and based on predefined activities in the risk management plan, the component is transferred to the outsource firm. There is no scrambling trying to identify and evaluate options when the event occurs.

8. Postdevelopment

A system is tested at various points in development to determine if expected functionality has been met. Testing begins at the unit level and continues until the complete system is tested in the production environment. An environment is hardware and software that is used to run the system and other systems. Typically, there is a development environment within which the developers build the system. There is a testing environment within which components of the systems are tested. There is a staging environment, which is a mirrored environment of the production environment and has all systems that are used to manage the facility. The staging environment is used to determine how the system performed with other systems in the organization. Finally, there is the production environment. The production environment consists of all the hardware and software the organization uses to operate.

Before a system is used by the organization, the system undergoes a set of progressive tests. These are:

- Unit test: A unit test, sometimes referred to as a component test, determines if a functional piece of the system meets specifications. Unit tests are conducted in either the development or test environment.

- Regression test: A regression test is performed when a defect occurs after a major change in the system is implemented that results in lost functionality. Typically, the regression test is conducted in the test environment.

- Integration test: The integration test tests all components of the system to determine if components work well together. Integration testing is usually performed in the test environment.

- Stress test: The stress test determines how the system will perform under a higher than expected volume of transactions. Some clinical project managers believe the stress test determines at what point the system will stop functioning. The stress test is performed in the test environment.

- Quality assurance test: The quality assurance test determines if the system meets standards of quality established by the organization. Typically, an internal group of quality testers or a vendor tries all possible scenarios for using the system, including scenarios that are unlikely to occur, with the goal of finding faults in the logic of the system. Quality assurance testing is performed in the test environment.

- User acceptance test: The user acceptance test determines if the system is acceptable to the project sponsor and stakeholders and is an element of the acceptance process (see Acceptance Process). The user acceptance test occurs in the test environment.

- System test: The system test is one of the final tests performed before the system is placed in the production environment. The goal of the system test is to determine if the system works well with other systems in the organization. The system test occurs in the staging environment. All systems except for the system being tested are systems currently running in the organization.

- Installation test: The installation test is the final test of the system before the organization uses the system. The installation test occurs immediately after the system is installed in the production environment and before the system goes live. The goal is to uncover any problems that may prevent the organization from using the system.

Acceptance Process

The acceptance process is the way that the project sponsor and stakeholders verify that the project meets expectations and performs according to specifications. The project began with a project chart, which is similar to a contract between the project sponsor and the clinical project manager that specifies terms within which the project is developed. The acceptance process is used by the project sponsor and the clinical project manager to assess if those terms were met.

The acceptance process begins during discussions about the project charter. The project chart should specify objective acceptance criteria that can be objectively measured by a user acceptance test. The actual user acceptance test should be developed shortly after the launch of the project and before development on the system begins.

There should be no surprises when the user performs the user acceptance test because the components of the test are known before development, enabling developers to ensure the system is able to pass the test. That is, developers perform the user acceptance test long before the acceptance test is performed by the user. Any defects are identified and fixed by developers.

There should be transparency during development of the system The project sponsor and stakeholders should participate in development. For example, a focus group of stakeholders should view and interact with screens during development to assess the accessibility and feasibility of the screens. Likewise, a focus group should participate in a walkthrough of processing logic and help design reports.

When development is completed and the system has passed the integrated and quality assurance tests, stakeholders can put the system through the user acceptance test. Typically, the user acceptance test involves common and uncommon scenarios based on daily activities. Stakeholders provide the testers and the site for testing. The user acceptance test is in the form of a script that contains routines and data used to test the system. Furthermore, the user acceptance test has expected outcomes, enabling the tester to enter the specified test data and compare the results with the expected outcomes. Defects may occur during the user acceptance test, requiring the developer to fix the problems and run the system through the same battery of tests again.

NURSING ALERT

The user acceptance test should be conducted at various locations throughout the organization to assess whether or not the location will impact the use of the system. For example, the facility may use Wi-Fi to connect computers to the network. There may be dead spots in some areas of the facility preventing a computer from connecting to the network.

Migration

After the project sponsor and stakeholders accept the system, the clinical project manager develops a migration plan to move the system into the production environment. The migration plan must consider:

- Conversation of existing data, if necessary.
- The effect migration will have on the organization.
- Operational constraints such as the effort required to migrate the system.
- Deciding criteria for a successful migration.
- Developing and implementing the installation test.
- The level of business disruption that is acceptable.
- The latitude to adjust the go live date.

The clinical project manager must work with the project sponsor and stakeholders to decide on the best migration strategy for the organization. There are general two migration strategies. These are:

- Gradual: A gradual migration occurs when the system is introduced to a portion of the organization at a time, usually beginning with the unit that would be least affected if problem arises with the system. Likewise, there is a gradual conversion of data from the existing system to the new system.
- All at once: The all-at-once migration strategy requires the entire organization to use the new system. The old system is turned off, and the new system is turned on. All data is converted before the changeover.
- Hybrid: The hybrid strategy requires the entire organization to use the new system; however, only recent data is converted to the new system at launch. Older data is gradually converted to the new system.
- Parallel: The parallel migration strategy requires that both the old and new system work at the same time. New data is entered into and processed by both systems. The clinical project manager and the project sponsor compare results. When the project sponsor is comfortable that the new system is producing acceptable results, the old system is turned off.

Close Out the Project

When the system is implemented, the clinical project manager and the project team close out the project. Initially, they gather and reflect on success and failures that occurred during development of the project. This is commonly referred to as "lessons learned" and is used to better manage future projects.

Documents that pertain to the project are archived so the information can be used as reference for revisions of the system or when developing a new system.

NURSING ALERT

Successful aspects of the project plan can be incorporated into a project template in Microsoft Project. The template can be used for a similar project, giving the clinical project manager a head start on planning the next project.

---

9. Agile Project Management

Not all clinical informatics project are as large and complex as implementing an electronic medical records system that requires a detailed project plan that specifies what needs to be done and when and by whom. Many projects that will be assigned to a nurse informatics specialist are relatively small and less complex and require a different project management methodology called Agile project management.

Agile project management is a way to organize and manage small, routine projects that require relatively small project teams of specialists who require general—not detailed—direction from the clinical project manager. General direction means that resources are told that a task must be performed. Resources determine subtasks, duration, and what other resources are required to perform the task. There is no formal project plan.

Let's say that a computer and printer need to be installed on a unit to print medication administration records during a power outage. The printer is directly connected to the computer, and the computer is connected to the eMAR system over the network. Every 2 hours, a printable copy of each patient's eMAR is loaded into the computer's hard drive. Both the computer and the printer are powered by the backup power supply.

The nurse informatics specialist makes the request to MIS. A technician is assigned the task. She assesses the unit, determines where the computer and printer should be located, arranges with the electrician to run the necessary wiring, acquires the computer and printer, and makes sure all subtasks are performed. The technician and other resources know what has to be done and how to do it.

Agile Method

The Agile methodology focuses on small batches of tasks that require intense collaboration of team members and stakeholders in face-to-face communication. The team is self-organizing. That is, the team sees the problem and determines what has to be done and who should solve the problem. Typically, each team member has a primary and one or more secondary skillsets. Team members are cross-functional and can step into multiple roles as required.

For example, one member may be primarily a clinical systems analyst and secondarily has some proficiency with computer hardware or can coordinate activities with stakeholders. The team adapts to change and responds to needs quickly.

Each small batch of tasks is revisited throughout the project as new needs are identified. The goal is to deliver a small batch of task and then continuously improve those batches to deliver quality results in the short time frame.

The project manager provides light-touch leadership. That is, each team member is empowered to learn about the problem, determine solutions, and engage stakeholders directly without experiencing the structure and constraints familiar with structure project management. Conversations between a team member and a stakeholder are likely to elicit new needs that can be brought back to the team and addressed based on the priority of the need.

The objective is to develop small features at a time from a work list called a focus board. The small feature is ready use, which is referred to as a product-ready deliverable. Small features are continuously integrated addressing the larger need of stakeholders.

The Focus Board

Stakeholders' needs are identified and entered into a focus board. The focus board can be a large flip chart or one or more white boards placed in a common area so every team member can view them at any time. The focus board is divided into three columns: To Do, In Progress, and Done (Table 5–1). An entry on the focus board is called a story (also referred to as a churn). A story is a brief narrative that describes a need such as to install a downtime computer and printer as illustrated in Table 5–1.

Notice that no tasks or resources are listed in the focus board. The Agile project team knows what needs to be done and how to do it. The team will acquire additional resources as needed to address the need. The team talks with stakeholders to determine priority and then works on the story with the highest priority.

NURSING ALERT

The focus board can list subtasks such as assessing requirements for installation of the downtime computer and printer, installing wiring, and installing the network connection.

TABLE 5–1 Focus Board Example

To Do	In Progress	Done
Install a downtime computer and printer for the eMAR system in Unit A7		

The Scrum

Agile project management uses the rugby approach. In rugby, the game is restarted after each minor infraction using a scrum. Players from both teams form a collective huddle with their arms interlocking their bodies. The ball is thrown inside the huddle, and each team member tries to recover the ball. Each team tries to go the distance to score a goal; however, the situation on the field can change at any moment, requiring the team to restart the game.

A similar situation exists with smaller, routine projects. Initially, stakeholders describe a need in general terms. Requirements are not fully defined. Furthermore, stakeholders are likely to change the need throughout the project. The Agile project team begins with a scrum working on the initial request. When a change occurs, the Agile project team stops, reassesses, and starts another scrum. The team's focus is on fast delivery of emerging requirements and then modifying delivered results to conform to the new requirements.

Sprint

A sprint is the basic unit of development in an Agile project and has a fixed duration such as 1 week, which is referred to as a time box. Sprints can be as long as 1 month. The priority item on the focus board is worked on during a sprint. If requirements are not completed, then the item is returned to the focus board and becomes the focus of another sprint.

For example, the technician might have completed a requirements analysis to install a backup computer and printer in Unit A7 during a sprint. Other steps remain open and can be performed during another sprint.

> **NURSING ALERT**
>
> Priorities can change between sprints, requiring the team to focus on completing an item different from the incomplete item of the previous sprint. For example, the team temporarily leaves the request to install a backup computer and printer in Unit A7 to a different sprint.

Sprint Planning Meeting

The sprint planning meeting is an 8-hour meeting held at the beginning of a sprint. The first 4 hours is spent reviewing work completed and presented to stakeholders and work that remains incomplete. The team determines what went well during the sprint and things that need to be improved during the next sprint. The backlog of items on the focus board is their priority.

The remaining 4 hours is spent planning the next sprint. That is, what work has to be done and identify the work that is likely to be accomplished during the sprint, giving the amount of effort required to perform the work. Each member of the team agrees to an assignment based on the priorities, and then the sprint begins.

Daily Scrum

The Agile project team meets daily at the same time in the same location to hold a team meeting called the daily scrum. The meeting lasts no more than 15 minutes, and everyone stands at the meeting. Each member is asked three questions. These are:

- What have you done since yesterday?
- What are you planning to do today?
- Are there any impediments in your way?

The focus of the meeting is to place the responsibility for planning and accomplishing daily activities on each team member. Furthermore, each team member is encouraged to ask for assistance when something impedes the team member's capability to deliver the result.

Backlog Grooming

Backlog grooming is the process of reviewing items on the focus board. The review process involves dividing large stories into smaller stories and refining the requirements of stakeholders to create more manageable stories. Stories are not broken into tasks and subtasks. The backlog grooming should take no more than 1 hour. The entire team participates in backlog grooming.

> **NURSING ALERT**
>
> There can be multiple of Agile teams, each working on different sets of items that either overlap or require integration. In this situation, a representative of each team forms a cluster. The cluster addresses mutual issues.

The Agile Project Team

The Agile project team consists of:

- Scrum master: The scrum master facilitates the scrum, removes impediments to completing stories, and keeps the team's focus on sprints by enforcing rules and buffering the team from distractions. Although the role of the scrum master has similarities to that of a project manager or team leader, the scrum master does not take on a leadership role.

- The team: The Agile team consists of up to nine members who have cross-functional skills and are responsible for delivering work at the end of each sprint.

- Product owner: The project owner represents stakeholders who requested the work. The project owner writes stories, prioritizes stories, and adds stories to the focus board. The project owner also ensures that the Agile team delivers value to stakeholders.

- Stakeholder: A stakeholder identifies a need for the organization and requests that that need be addressed by the Agile project team. The stakeholder receives deliverables and either accepts and implements the deliverable into the organization's workflow or rejects the deliverable, requiring the Agile project team to rework the item. The stakeholder has no formal role in the project and is rarely involved in the Agile process.

CASE STUDY

CASE 1

The chief operating officer of the healthcare facility assigns you as the clinical project manager for implementing the healthcare facility's first electronic medical records system. The electronic medical records system replaces paper charts and many manual processes required for processing those charts. This is the first major project for the healthcare facility in 3 years. The chief operating officer trusts you but wants comfort that you can address her concerns. She asks you the following questions. What are your best responses?

QUESTION 1. How do you estimate the cost of the project?
ANSWER: The cost is determined using a bottom-up approach. First all tasks are identified; then duration and dependencies are established. Resources are identified and assigned to each task. Each resource has an associated cost, and therefore the estimated cost for each task can be calculated. Additional costs such as licensing fees and upgrades to the healthcare facility's infrastructure and computers are added to the calculation. A contingency of about 15% is then added to arrive at the estimated cost.

QUESTION 2. Do you need a project plan because the healthcare facility is acquiring the electronic medical records application from a vendor?
ANSWER: Yes. Although the vendor is providing the application, many tasks and resources are necessary for the healthcare facility to implement the electronic medical records application. These tasks must be identified and included in a formal project plan to ensure that all tasks are completed on time in support of the vendor's delivery of the electronic medical records application.

QUESTION 3. How can we measure the performance of the project?
ANSWER: The project plan is divided into deliverables and milestones, each projected to be realized by a specific date. The chief operating officer, administrators, project sponsor, and stakeholders as well as the project team will use deliverables and milestones as a measurement of performance.

QUESTION 4. Should the vendor be responsible for managing the project?
ANSWER: No. Implementation of the electronic medical records application is the responsibility of the healthcare facility. The vendor's contribution is part of the project. There are workflows and operational considerations, in addition to use of the healthcare facility's own resources that are involved in the implementation of the electronic medical records application. Therefore, the healthcare facility should manage the project with the advice and cooperation of the vendor.

FINAL CHECK-UP

1. **What is the purpose of a project charter?**
    A. A project charter specifies responsibilities for stakeholders.
    B. A project charter specifies responsibilities for each project team member.
    C. A project charter specifies all tasks associated with the project.
    D. A project charter specifies what the project manager is to deliver and the terms under which the project manager will manage the project.

2. **What is a task?**
    A. A task is something someone does.
    B. A task is an action that has a beginning and an end that produces a result.
    C. A task is an element of the project charter.
    D. A task is an element of a milestone.

3. **What is a milestone?**
    A. A milestone is a reportable finding to stakeholders by the project manager.
    B. A milestone is the length of time the project teams works on the project.
    C. A milestone is an output of an action.
    D. A milestone is a measurement of significant progress.

4. **What is duration?**
    A. Duration is the length of time resources work on a task plus elapsed time.
    B. Duration is the length of the project.
    C. Duration is the time necessary to create the project charter.
    D. Duration is the time required to begin the project.

5. **What is the purpose of a resource list?**

   A. The resource list is used by the finance department to pay employees who work on the project.

   B. The resource list is a list of assignments for each resource working on the project.

   C. The resource list contains available resources, time available to work on the project, and costs associated with the resource.

   D. The resource lists contains the rationale for employing each resources on the project.

6. **What is resource overallocation?**

   A. Allocating too many resources to a task.

   B. Allocating a resource to tasks beyond the time that the resource is available to work on the project.

   C. Allocating a shared resource to the project.

   D. Allocating stakeholders to tasks on the project.

7. **When would Agile project methodology be used on a project?**

   A. Agile project methodology is used for relatively small, complex projects that can be accomplished by a team of up to nine members who are cross-functional.

   B. Agile project methodology is used for relatively small, routine, less complex projects that can be accomplished by a team of up to nine members who are cross-functional.

   C. Agile project methodology is used for relatively large, complex projects that can be accomplished by a team of up to nine members who are cross-functional.

   D. Agile project methodology is used for projects that require flexibility.

8. **What is the importance of a sprint in an Agile project?**

   A. A sprint is an activity performed by an Agile project team to groom the backlog of stories on the focus board.

   B. A sprint is an activity performed by an Agile project team to set priorities of stories.

   C. A sprint is a unit of work that lasts a fixed duration such as 1 week but can be upwards to 1 month.

   D. A sprint is a unit of work that lasts a variable duration such as 1 week but can be upwards to 1 month.

9. **When should the user acceptance test be developed?**

   A. At the halfway point in the project
   B. Near the end of the project
   C. At the start of the project
   D. Before the project begins

10. **What is the purpose of the risk management plan?**

   A. A risk management plan identifies risks associated with project development and defines how the nurse informatics project manager will address each risk.
   B. A risk management plan identifies risks associated with the clinical application and defines how each risk will be addressed.
   C. A risk management plan identifies risks associated with the healthcare facility and defines how each risk will be addressed.
   D. A risk management plans identifies risks associated with the healthcare industry and defines how each risk will be addressed.

CORRECT ANSWERS AND RATIONALES

1. D. A project charter specifies what the project manager is to deliver and the terms under which the project manager will manage the project.
2. B. A task is an action that has a beginning and an end that produces a result.
3. D. A milestone is a measurement of significant progress.
4. A. Duration is the length of time resources work on a task plus elapsed time.
5. C. The resource list contains available resources, time available to work on the project, and costs associated with the resource.
6. B. Allocating a resource to tasks beyond the time that the resource is available to work on the project.
7. B. Agile project methodology is used for relatively small, routine, less complex projects that can be accomplished by a team of up to nine members who are cross-functional.
8. C. A sprint is a unit of work that lasts a fixed duration such as 1 week but can be upwards to 1 month.
9. C. At the start of the project.
10. A. The risk management plans identifies risks associated with project development and defines how the nurse informatics project manager will address each risk.

chapter 6

Clinical Informatics Team Management

LEARNING OBJECTIVES

1. Project team management
2. Conflict resolution
3. Group dynamics
4. Effective communication
5. Management techniques

KEY TERMS

Effective listening	SBAR
Mediation	Shared values
OODA loop model	Stages of adoption
Project sponsor	Steering committee
RACI chart	Team-driven planning
Rapid planning	Virtual project teams
Real-time planning	Work groups
Relationship capital	

1. Project Team Management

The project manager is the manager of the project and the project team. The project manager is also the facilitator of the project, coordinating project activities with the **project sponsor,** stakeholders, and the project team to ensure that expectations are well defined and objectively measurable and that the project team delivers a system that meets the expectations of the project sponsor and stakeholders.

The project team consists of various numbers of professionals with different skillsets. Many team members have cross-functional expertise, enabling them to contribute in multiple ways to the project. The number of team members and their skillsets vary depending on the nature of the project. Some members are on the team for the length of the project, but others join and leave the team after they make their contribution to the project.

The project manager is the single leader of the team who makes decisions about the project with advice from members of the team, stakeholders, and the project sponsor. The project manager uses open problem-solving techniques to address challenges that arise during the project. Open problem-solving techniques require that all problems be shared among team members, encouraging each to help solve problems. The team has collective goals and is mutually accountable for meeting expectations.

Work Group

The team is divided into **work groups** depending on the needs of the project. A work group is a subset of the team that has a clear, measurable objective that addresses a portion of the project's objective. The work group has a work group leader who takes on many of the project manager's roles and responsibilities related to the work group. The work group is mutually accountable for achieving the work group's goal. A work group can remain intact throughout the project and collectively work on different aspects of the project. Alternatively, a work group can be assembled to achieve one goal. After the goal is met, work group members disperse later to a different work group with different members of the project team.

Project Management Role

The project manager has many roles in a project. The foremost role is as a leader who takes control of the project and manages the project from inception of an idea to implementing an actual system. Key elements of project management are:

- Effective planning: Effective planning is the ability to decompose an idea into tasks and organize tasks into a detailed plan that clearly defines steps needed to make the idea into reality.

- Define roles and responsibilities: Defining roles and responsibilities is a management task of identifying and organizing resources that will perform tasks specified in the project plan. The project manager decides who does what and when each activity is performed.

- Define work rules: A work rule provides a framework within which resources perform an activity. Work rules are defined based on constraints specified in the project charter and policies and procedures of the organization. Work rules do not tell a resource how to perform an activity, however. The resource has the flexibility to perform an activity as long as the performance complies with the work rules.

- Manage conflicts: Expectations, a detailed project plan, and work rules combined with flexibility of a resource to perform an activity can cause conflicts. No project plan is perfect. No work rule is perfect. And at times, expectations may not be realistic. A key role and responsibility of a project manager is to manage conflict.

RACI Chart

A common technique to organize the project and the project team—and reduce opportunity for conflict—is to develop a **RACI chart** for the project. A RACI chart defines:

- Responsibility: Each task is assigned to a resource or a group of resources who is responsible for completing the task.

- Accountability: A resource is assigned accountability for delivery of the task and that the task meets expectations.
- Consulted: Resources who must be consulted about how a task is performed are identified by the project manager.
- Informed: The project manager identifies resources that must be kept informed on the progress of developing the task.

For example, a work group is responsible for developing specifications for an electronic medical record administration record (eMAR). The project manager, the work group leader, and members of the work group are accountable that the specifications are developed and meet expectations. Stakeholders must be consulted during the development of specifications for the eMAR. The project manager and project sponsor must be kept informed about progress developing the specifications.

Developing a RACI chart for each task ensures that those involved in the task know their roles and responsibilities.

2. Conflict Resolution

Conflict within a project cannot be avoided; however, the project manager can take steps to minimize opportunity for conflict to arise. These steps include:

- Keeping lines of communication open: Free flow of accurate information is critical to avoid conflict, and information can only flow if lines of communication among the project team and the project manager remain open during the duration of the project.
- One-on-one conversations: The project manager should converse individually with each member of the project team to identify potential conflicts and to ensure that each member is working with accurate information.
- Hold regular staff meetings: Staff meetings provide a forum for exploration and discussion on challenges faced by the project team and possible strategies to meet those challenges. A staff meeting is also the place where issues are clarified (see Group Dynamics).
- Participation in the decision process: A person who participates in a decision develops a feeling of ownership in the decision. Conflicts between the person's opinions and recommendations and the decision are resolved if the person helps to make the decision.
- Feedback: Each team member should be encouraged to speak openly and honestly during one-on-one conversations and during meetings (see Group Dynamics).

- Test the waters: Discuss potential changes with each member of the project team, stakeholders, and the project sponsor recommending the change. The project manager will learn about and can address potential conflicts before the recommendation is put forth.

- Make small changes: Conflicts decrease when change is made incrementally.

- Be honest: Truthfulness can avoid conflicts. A person may not embrace what is said but can appreciate that the person made an honest statement.

Mediate a Conflict

When conflicts arise, the project manager takes on the role of mediator. A mediator's role is to create an environment where parties to the conflict can resolve their differences. Facts in dispute tend to overshadow facts that are in agreement. Parties tend to become emotional over the conflict, which clouds their rational thought process.

The project manager must remain calm and be a neutral party to the conflict. Give an hour or two as a cooling-off period so that the parties can regain composure. Call a meeting at a neutral place away from the flow of traffic so that there will be no interruptions. The goal is to have parties revisit the issue that caused the conflict with an open mind. The project manager must focus attention on the issue and not on the personalities of the parties.

Begin by helping the parties identify facts that are in agreement. Use either a legal pad or a white board and write a list of facts not in dispute. This list is usually much longer than the list of disputed facts. An objective is to make this list visibly long.

Next, help the parties identify facts that are in dispute. Make a list of those facts alongside the list of facts in agreement. This list tends to be small. An objective is to make this list visibly short.

Looking at both lists should make it obvious that the parties are in agreement on everything except for a very few facts. The project manager should reinforce this observation by glancing at the lists and saying, "Looks like your differences are small when compared with everything."

Next, dissect each fact in dispute into elements. List elements of each fact that are in agreement and list elements in dispute in a separate list. Place these lists to the right of the list of facts in dispute. The list of elements of the disputed fact tends to be longer than the elements in dispute. The process of identifying elements that are disputed helps to place the conflict in perspective for the parties. Each party can see that they agree on most things, including a lot of elements in the disputed fact.

At the end of this exercise, there is a list of a few facts that parties agreed are in dispute. The project manager then focuses everyone's attention on the first disputed fact. Each party is invited to explain their position while others are asked to listen and avoid interruptions. Each party is then invited to respond.

It is important for the project manager to listen carefully to each position and counterposition in an effort to identify common ground. The project manager should restate each position and opposing argument in a calm, deliberate voice, saying, "Here's what I heard you say. . . ." Give each party time to correct your understanding.

Summarize the status of the disagreement and open the floor to possible solutions. Help each side think through the proposal by exploring the advantages and disadvantages and provide a reality check. A reality check separates theory from practice and helps the parties focus on a realistic solution to the conflict.

The **mediation** process provides parties with a realistic view of the conflict and helps them focus on finding an acceptable solution. Parties may agree to disagree, but they will come up with a way to continue to work as a team.

3. Group Dynamics

Although we tend to think of a group as a cohesive entity, a group is actually composed of individuals, each of whom has a personality, beliefs, and a way of interacting with others. This is referred to as group dynamics. A project manager who facilitates meetings needs to be aware of group dynamics and use the dynamics of the group to help the group achieve the meeting goals.

Each participant in a group naturally takes on one or more definable roles within the group during the course of the meeting. None of these roles are assigned to them by the project manager. Instead, each group member is drawn into the role by changing dynamics of others who attend the meeting.

Here are the roles commonly found in a group:

- Initiator or contributor: The initiator or contributor proposes various ways the group can achieve the group's goal. The person has a positive, can-do attitude.

- Information seeker: The information seeker evaluates information presented at the meeting by the project manager and others to assess if the information is relevant, asks for clarification, and then determines information that is missing and necessary to address the group's goal.

- Information giver: The information giver is an authority of the subject matter and provides the group with factual information.

- Opinion seeker: An opinion seeker encourages everyone in the group to voice an opinion.

- Opinion giver: An opinion giver offers an opinion to the group.

- Elaborator: An elaborator embellishes on ideas of others in the group by providing facts and voicing the consequences of a proposal.

- Coordinator: A coordinator consolidates various suggestions into one cohesive suggestion.

- Orienter: An orienter brings the discussion back on track by summarizing information that has been discussed.

- Evaluator or critic: The evaluator or critic assesses the reasonableness of a suggestion and considers when the suggestion is achievable.

- Energizer: The energizer stimulates the group into action by focusing on progress made toward the goal.

- Procedural technician: The procedural technician makes all arrangements for the meeting.

- Recorder: The recorder keeps the minutes of the meeting and distributes minutes after the meeting.

Positive Roles

Some group members take on a role that helps the group move toward the goal. These roles are referred to as positive roles. The project manager should encourage group members whose efforts foster the group to work cohesively to reach a viable outcome.

Here are positive roles within a group:

- Encourager: The encourager voices support for group members whose participation moves the group along toward reaching a goal.

- Harmonizer: The harmonizer defuses tension by finding common ground among competing opinions to keep the discussion positive (see Mediate a Conflict).

- Compromiser: The compromiser changes a position to come closer to an opposition position to move the group toward the goal.

- Gatekeeper or expediter: The gatekeeper or expediter keeps communication among group members flowing by encouraging quiet members to voice an opinion and limiting participation by group members who dominate the conversation.

- Observer or commentator: The observer or commentator gives group members feedback on how well the group is functioning to reach the goal.

- Follower: The follower listens but does not contribute to the group discussion and has not voiced an opinion on the group's conclusion except to go along with the group's decision.

Disruptive Roles

Some group members disrupt the cohesiveness of the group and progress toward reaching a consensus. This is referred to as a disruptive role. The project manager must take steps to reduce the effectiveness of group members who are disruptive to the group.

Here are disruptive roles:

- Aggressor: The aggressor belittles, insults, and personally attacks one or more members of the group.
- Blocker: The blocker objects to every opinion and does not put forward an original suggestion.
- Recognition seeker: The recognition seeker focuses attention on himself by exaggerating his importance and expertise.
- Self-confessor: The self-confessor expresses personal issues during the meeting.
- Playboy or playgirl: The playboy or playgirl sees the meeting as a way to avoid working and focuses on personal interactions with colleagues.
- Dominator: The dominator controls the meeting and group members, although he is not the project manager.
- Help seeker: The help seeker poses as being helpless and looks for sympathy from group members.
- Special interest pleader: The special interest pleader conceals his opinion and voices stereotypical views that he thinks are acceptable by group members.

4. Effective Communication

Communication is a critical component of every project because communication is the vehicle that establishes expectations. Expectations are outcomes that the project sponsor, stakeholders, and members of the project team have about the project. Some clinical project managers consider expectations as the goal line. If expectations are met, then the project is considered successful. If expectations are not met, then the project has failed.

Let's say that the clinical project manager tells stakeholders that all light-bulbs on a unit will be replaced in 20 minutes. The clinical project manager has set expectations. Technicians who replace lightbulbs know that the task, given the number of technicians assigned to the task, will take 60 minutes based on their experience changing lightbulbs. However, it takes 60 minutes to change lightbulbs on the unit. The clinical project manager's expectations are not met, so stakeholders consider the effort a failure.

The problem was with lack of communication between the clinical project manager and the resource assigned to perform the task. As a result, this small project failed. Yet expectations would have been met if the clinical project manager stated at the onset that changing lightbulbs on the unit would take 60 minutes.

NURSING ALERT

All clinical projects are completed on time and on budget. Estimates of when the project will be completed and the projected budgets are wrong if the project seems to not deliver on time and over budget. We judge success by expectations established by the plan. If expectations are wrong, we tend to blame the reality of performing the tasks rather than the estimate.

Identify the Audience

Each message should be designed for the needs of the intended audience to ensure that the message is accurately received. Take, for example, an eMAR system. The chief operating officer (COO) of the facility is interested in compliance with regulatory requirements and qualifying for government reimbursement for the project. The federal government reserved $19 billion of reimbursement funds that can be dispersed to facilities to adopt and effectively use electronic medical records. This is commonly referred to as meaningful use. In contrast, nurses are focused on ease of use and whether or not eMAR will disrupt their effective workflow on the unit.

A good communicator identifies each unique stakeholder such as the COO, vice presidents, directors, assistant directors, unit managers, nurses, pharmacy, and others who are affected by or are interested in the clinical project.

Next, the needs of each stakeholder are assessed. The clinical project manager must identify why the stakeholder needs to receive the message. There are four reasons why a clinical project manager communicates with a stakeholder. These are:

- Responsible: The stakeholder is responsible for one or more aspects of the clinical project. That is, the stakeholder must contribute to the clinical project. For example, the clinical project manager and the project team are responsible for the design and implementation of the eMAR system.

- Accountable: A stakeholder is accountable when the stakeholder is exposed to consequences if the project fails to meet expectations even though the stakeholder has limited or no active role in the project. For example, the vice president of management information systems (MIS) is accountable for the successful implementation of an eMAR system, yet other stakeholders are responsible for the design and implementation of the eMAR system.

- Consulted: A stakeholder who is a content expert is consulted by the clinical project manager, project team, and possibly other stakeholders throughout the project. However, the content expert is not responsible or accountable for the outcome of the project.

- Informed: The clinical project manager needs to keep the COO, vice presidents, director of nursing, assistant director of nurse, nurse managers, and nursing staff abreast of the project status. These stakeholders do not directly participate in the project.

NURSING ALERT

The role of a stakeholder may change throughout the course of the project; therefore, the manner in which the clinical project sponsor communicates with them must also change.

A RACI (responsible, accountable, consulted, informed) chart (Table 6–1) can be used to assess the types of communication that is needed for each activity. It is best to informally assign individual stakeholders to a group that has

TABLE 6–1 The RACI Chart Helps to Analyze Communication as the Need of Stakeholders

Activity	COO	VP MIS	Exec Nurse	Directors	Assistant Directors	Unit Managers	Nurses	Project Team
Activity 1	I	A	C	I	I	C	C	R
Activity 2	I	A	C	I	C	C	I	R
Activity 3	I	A	C	I	I	C	I	R

COO = chief operating officer; MIS = management information systems; RACI = responsible, accountable, consulted, informed; VP = vice president.

similar communications needs. Limit customized individual communication to those who don't fit into a group such as the COO and executive nurse.

Before composing the communication, identify the purpose of sending the communication. What is your reason for communicating with them, and what action do you want them to take? Keep in mind that stakeholders receive a lot of emails, especially those high in the chain of command. Stakeholders want the clinical project manager to tell them something they do not know and tell them why they should know it. Answer these questions in the subject line of the email and you have a good chance that the email will be read.

Communications Plan

Give careful thought to what needs to be communicated and how it will be communicated throughout the life cycle of the project. This is commonly referred to as the communications plan. Develop the communications plan by assessing the communications expectations of stakeholders. The best way to do this is to ask each key stakeholder:

- What information does the stakeholder need throughout the project?
- When does the stakeholder need the information?
- How would the stakeholder like to receive the information?

For example, the COO may request the vice president of MIS to provide weekly updates of all mission critical projects in a weekly email. The update should only include indicators if each project is on time and on budget and one sentence for each project explaining exceptions.

In contrast, the executive nurse wants communication to be delivered at a meeting with key stakeholders held every other week during the project life cycle. The invitation to the meeting should contain an agenda, and attendees are expected to assist in decision making for each agenda item.

The clinical project manager can easily formulate a framework for effectively communicating with all stakeholders after the assessment is completed and the communications plan is developed. As a result, the clinical project manager will not be overwhelmed with keeping stakeholders' information, and stakeholders will not be overwhelmed receiving unnecessary messages.

NURSING ALERT

Each activity in the project should have a clearly defined goal and a clearly defined metric used to measure progress toward achieving the goal. The metric can be used to give stakeholders a snapshot of the progress that is being made to achieve the goal.

The Skills of Communication

The clinical project manager knows the content that needs to be shared with stakeholders; however, the formulation and transmission of those thoughts can be miscommunicated unless careful thought is given to the communication itself.

Shared symbols are the foundation of communication. A shared symbol is a word, a phrase, body language, or other means that is used to communicate that has the same meaning to the sender and receiver of the communication. For example, the acronym eMAR stands for electronic medical administration record. eMAR and electronic medical administration record are both symbols that are used in communication. The person sending the communication must be sure that the receiver of the communication understands the meaning of eMAR and electronic medical administration record; otherwise, the sender's thoughts are miscommunicated.

At the beginning of a project, the clinical project manager should develop a glossary of terms (shared symbols) that will be used in communication throughout the project. The glossary should contain clinical terms, MIS terms, and terms that are unique to the facility such as abbreviations for units. Stakeholders can refer to the glossary to either formulate communication or interpret communication.

The method of communication can impact whether or not thoughts are communicated accurately. Some communication methods provide immediate feedback, enabling the sender to identify miscommunication that can be corrected immediately. Other communication methods provide little or no feedback, exposing the sender and receiver to the risk of miscommunication. Different types of communication include:

- In person: When speaking with someone, we can easily read body language to have an inkling of whether or not the message is being received accurately. Both parties have the opportunity to ask questions and clarify any misunderstanding.

- Telephone: Communication via telephone also enables parties to ask questions and clarify misunderstandings; however, there is no opportunity to read body language, and therefore there remains a risk of undetected miscommunication.

- Written: Written communication has a high risk for miscommunication for a number of reasons. First, the sender is never sure that the communication was read in its entirety—or read at all. There is no feedback that the message was actually communicated. Furthermore, the receiver of the message must make an effort to contact the sender for clarification.

- Email: Email has the same risk as the written method of communication for miscommunication. In addition, there is a risk of creating a misperception. For example, words in capital letters might be perceptive as "electronic shouting" when it might merely be caused by mistyping, especially because emails are at times sent via mobile devices.

> **NURSING ALERT**
>
> Attempt to minimize distraction when delivering your message. Tell the receiver why it is important to listen or read in your opening sentence; otherwise, the receiver is likely to become distracted.

SBAR

SBAR is a communication framework developed by the military in World War II to focus a leader on information needed to make a decision quickly. SBAR has since been adopted by the healthcare industry as the framework to communicate effectively and efficiently among staff.

SBAR stands for situation, background, assessment, and recommendations and is the format that clinical project managers should use when constructing a message to stakeholders. First state the reason for the communication in the opening sentence. Next briefly give the background as to what has led up to the issue. Provide a brief assessment of options available to resolve or mitigate the issue. Next put forth your recommendation. For example:

- Situation: The clinical analyst resigned today, and this will potentially place us 3 months behind on the eMAR implementation.

- Background: The clinical analyst is moving across the country because his significant other is relocating due to employment. The clinical analyst was in the process of using the vendor's tool to modify the eMAR application to meet our needs.

- Assessment: There are two options available. Hiring a new clinical analyst will take 3 months before the clinical analyst is up to speed on making the necessary modifications. Alternatively, the task can be outsourced to the vendor because our specifications have already been developed. This will cost $10,000 and put us 2 weeks behind schedule.

- Recommendation: I suggest we outsource the task to the vendor because this will enable us to remain on schedule and realize reimbursements sooner than if the project was delayed for 3 months.

Notice in this example that the decision maker is focused on the recommendation and not focused on understanding the problem and exploring alternative solutions to the problem. All that work was done by the clinical project manager and presented in a consistent message.

Barriers to Effective Communication

In addition to shared symbols and methods of communication, there are other barriers to effective communication that the clinical project manager should consider when developing a communication plans for the project. These are:

- Personalities: A personality is an emotional, attitudinal, and behavioral response pattern of an individual to an activity that can interfere with effective communication. At times the sender's and receiver's personalities can clash, focusing attention on each other rather than on the message being communicated. The clinical project manager should assess each stakeholder's personality and find a communication method that complements the personality. For example, written communication might be more appropriate than face-to-face communication if the clinical project manager's personality clashes with the stakeholder.

- Skills: Successful communication requires basic reading, writing, and listening skills. Lack of these skills can block communication. This is particularly concerning when English is a sender's or receiver's second language if the receiver is embarrassed to ask that the message be restated in terms that are more easily understood by the receiver. The clinical project manager should anticipate potential problems related to basic skills and then communicate using a method that reduces the effect of this barrier. For example, a walkthrough of a system using screenshots or the actual application can effectively communicate even if there is a language barrier.

- Defensive: The stakeholder may find the project threatening to the stakeholder's position and therefore is not receptive to receiving the message. For example, a nurse comfortable with using the paper medical record administration record (MAR) might feel threatened with the eMAR because the nurse is uncomfortable using the computer. Any discussion of the eMAR places the nurse on the defensive. The clinical project manager should anticipate objections by stakeholders and then develop a communications plan to decrease the stakeholders' anxiety. For example, the clinical project manager may ask the nurse what aspect of his job he dislikes. The nurse may state that taking orders is challenging. The clinical project manager can respond by saying the pharmacy takes orders in the eMAR system. The eMAR system makes the nurse's job easier.

- Timing: Timing is everything when communicating a message to a stakeholder. The stakeholder must be in the right mindset to receive the message; otherwise, the stakeholder will not pay attention to the message. Finding the right time to deliver the message can be challenging. The clinical project manager should assess the period in the day when the stakeholder is most likely to be receptive to the message. For example, a clinical project manager may wait until 6 a.m. to send an email to the executive nurse, knowing that the executive nurse checks her emails at that hour before leaving for home. Also, the clinical project manager's email is likely to be at the top of the executive nurse's email inbox because there are few emails sent at that hour.

Stages of Adoption

Each stakeholder goes through an evaluation process before the stakeholder agrees with what the clinical project manager proposes. This evaluation process is referred to as **stages of adoption**. The challenge is that the clinical project manager has already completed the stages of adoption and is therefore sold on the idea; however, the idea still has to be sold to stakeholders. Therefore, the clinical project manager must focus on helping stakeholders work through each stage of adoption by providing information to complete each stage.

Here are the stages of adoption:

- Awareness: The stakeholder needs to be aware of a problem and that a solution exists. For example, the stakeholder must know the pitfalls of using a paper MAR and that those deficits do not exist in an eMAR system.

- Exploration: The stakeholder takes a superficial look at the proposed solution to determine if the proposal is viable. That is, the stakeholder may look up eMAR on the web to learn more about eMAR.

- Examination: Having decided for himself that eMAR may be a viable alternative, the stakeholder contacts colleagues at a facility that is using eMAR and ask for a walkthrough.

- Test: Now that the stakeholder is satisfied that eMAR is likely beneficial to the facility, the stakeholder logically tests the eMAR system under various scenarios. For example, the stakeholder asks how eMAR works in power outages or if a patient is in isolation. During this exercise, the stakeholder is trying to answer the question, "Why not adopt eMAR for the facility?"

- Adoption: The stakeholder agrees that the facility should adopt an eMAR system.

The clinical project manager should provide the stakeholder with websites that help the stakeholder explore the idea and contacts at facilities that have already adopted the idea, enabling the stakeholder to closely examine the idea. The clinical project manager should also provide the clinical project manager with a list of common concerns and how each is addressed. This helps the stakeholder through the test stage of adoption.

> **NURSING ALERT**
>
> Do not rush a stakeholder through the stages of adoption. Each stakeholder needs to work through the process himself.

Effective Listening

We learn more from listening than speaking. As a clinical project manager, it is critical that you develop **effective listening** techniques to gather as much information as you can to develop a successful project plan and manage stakeholder expectations.

Here are a few factors that break down barriers to listening:

- Always focus on what can be learned from the speaker rather than the speaker himself. The speaker maybe a poor communicator but has a valuable message to deliver.

- Maintain eye contact with speaker. This demonstrates that you are paying attention to the speaker.

- Avoid being distracted. Ignore ringing telephones and incoming text messages during the conversation. Some clinical project managers even lock the conference room door when the meeting begins to prevent interruptions.

- Make sure your body language expresses interest in what is being said. Face the speaker and relax.

- Give feedback during the conversation to demonstrate that you received the message. This also enables the speaker to correct any misperceptions.

- Ask probing questions but do not place the speaker in an embarrassing situation. Always give the speaker a way to save face. Let's say that the speaker spoke in error. You might respond, "I see" and say, "If I heard you correctly, you said . . ." and then restate the point correctly.

- Do not be afraid to slow down the presentation if the speaker is going too fast. You might ask, "If you don't mind, can we go over that last point again?"

- Be alert that the speaker may not fully understand the message himself. That is, the message may involve complex technical material that requires clarification by a context expert. Do not pressure the speaker for clarification. Instead, seek clarification from an appropriate party after the presentation.

Delivering Bad News

One of the most difficult jobs of a clinical project manager is to deliver bad news when expectations are not being met. This is an unpleasant situation for the clinical project manager, for the project team, and for others involved in the project. No one likes failure and the consequences that might come as a result of the failure. Breaking the bad news requires a communication plan so that the magnitude of the problem is known and focus can be directed to recovery.

Here are some techniques clinical project managers use to manage bad news:

- Do not become emotionally involved. Stay objective and do not take anything said to your heart.

- Take control over the situation and set the tone by speaking with confidence. Work toward developing a reasonable solution that minimizes exposure to potential problems.

- Fact find. Assess the impact of the problem on the project and operation of the healthcare facility. Do not be afraid to change direction.

- Avoid talking until your assessment is completed and you have a plan to address the problem.

- Give an objective appraisal of the situation. Do not minimize or overstate the situation.

- Explain the problem and explore options to remedy the problem. The goal is recovery, not assigning blame.

- Allow time for stakeholders to explore and understand the problem (see Stages of Adoption).

- Prepare a recommendation that includes tasks, duration, and costs necessary to fix the problem.

- Identify ways that the problem can be prevented from reoccurring.

- Maintain a high status—a leader—and keep an arm's length away from disputes. Make yourself appear to be a person who speaks objectively about the problem and can solve the problem.

- Initiate the solution, if possible, before bringing the issue before management. This enables you to say, "Here is the problem, and here is how we are fixing it." Management is usually more receptive to bad news if the clinical project manager has already taken steps to address the problem.

- Reestablish expectations. Identify what you expect from others to solve the problem and identify what management expects from you and your project team. Be flexible and do not be afraid to negotiate favorable expectations. Remember that expectations define success.

- Above all, make sure that the problem is fixed.

5. Management Techniques

The success of a clinical project is dependent on the nurse informatics specialist to gain and sustain commitment from the project team, administration, and clinicians throughout the healthcare facility. To achieve success, the nurse informatics specialist must:

- Establish trust and confidence by managing expectations and then meet those expectations. Success is defined by meeting expectations.

- Ensure that stakeholders receive value during development of the clinical project. Value is something that the stakeholder can appreciate throughout the course of the project rather than simply waiting until the project is delivered. For example, stakeholders can be brought into the decision process related to changes in clinical workflows or designs of screens.

- Unleash motivation and innovation in the project team. Team members must feel comfortable thinking out of the box and trying new, unproven approaches to solve problems confronting the project team.

- Have a commanding presence throughout the project, maintaining control during challenging periods and taking appropriate action to address problems.

Virtual Project Teams

The nursing informatics project manager should form a relatively small nuclear project team that is embellished by **virtual project teams**. A virtual project team consists of subject matter experts who join the project team to address a specific issue related to the subject matter. After the issue is resolved, the subject matter expert returns to normal duties.

Virtual project teams offer flexibility and reduced cost because the size of the team is scalable to the needs of the project at that moment in time. Issues can be addressed without increasing full-time equivalent positions on the clinical project team by temporarily reassigning existing staff to the project.

Many times virtual team members will work either part time on the project or on ad-hoc committees in the role of consultants.

> **NURSING ALERT**
>
> Float pool, part-time, and per diem employees are ideal candidates for membership in a virtual project team because they are likely to have flexible clinical assignments.

Virtual teams may have little or no loyalty to the project because they focus on one aspect of the project. They may share little experience and friendship with other virtual team members, and this might lead to limited trust. Therefore, the nurse informatics project manager needs to engage virtual team members and make them believe that they have a valued interest in the success of the entire project.

Shared Values

The success of a clinical project depends on **shared values** among members of the clinical project team and all stakeholders on the project. It is the responsibility of the nurse informatics project manager to encourage everyone involved in the project to adopt these values. These are:

- Trust: There must be mutual trust among the project team, the stakeholders, and the nurse informatics project manager otherwise, mistrust will perpetuate and build during the project presenting a high risk for failure.
- Openness: There must be free flow of information among the project team and stakeholders. All information should be presented factually without embellishment and without half-truths.
- Proactive: Each member of the project team and stakeholders must be proactive in identifying problems and coming up with solutions.
- Participative: Each member of the project team and stakeholders must have meaningful participation in the project. That is, each must help work toward completing the project.

Relationship Capital

Professional and informal relationships develop with colleagues throughout the nurse informatics specialist's career in the healthcare facility. Reputation with colleagues establishes creditability and trust. This relationship is referred to as **relationship capital** and can be used to effectively manage the project.

The relationship is referred to as capital because the relationship has intrinsic value. For example, the nurse informatics specialist may tell a stakeholder that an issue raised by the stakeholder is minor and will be resolved shortly. There is no evidence supporting the claim. If the stakeholder has a positive relationship with the nurse informatics specialists, then the stakeholder is likely to give the benefit of the doubt and consider the claim as true. However, the stakeholder will probably continue to be concerned and escalate the issue if a relationship does not exist.

In general, the more relationship capital a nurse informatics specialist has, the easier her job will be managing the project. However relationship capital diminishes each time the relationship is used to enlist support. That is, a stakeholder wants to see issues resolved and not simply that issues will be resolved sometime in the future.

Relationship capital is accumulated over time by delivering on promises and speaking the truth. If an issue will be resolved and is resolved, then the promise was kept, and relationship capital is received. If an issue will not be resolved and stakeholders are notified in advance, then relationship capital is received because the nurse informatics specialist spoke the truth—even if the stakeholder did not like the truth.

A goal of the nurse informatics specialist is to build relationships—and relationship capital—with stakeholders, administrators, clinicians, and each member of the project team.

Team-Driven Planning

Project planning should be a collaborative effort to ensure all concerns are considered and accurately addressed in the plan. Team members, stakeholders, and subject matter experts should participate in planning. Experts from different background have a greater capacity for exploring and devising a strategy for handling the complexity of the project.

Some researchers believe that the benefit of **team-driven planning** is development of a more accurate plan than using a traditional project management methodology. Traditional project management methodology requires the project manager to take on the expert's role in the project rather than be a facilitator of experts, which is the foundation of team-driven planning. A drawback of using team-driven planning is the influence group dynamics has on building a consensus (see Group Dynamics), which might result in developing an inaccurate plan. In addition, the plan is devised by a committee, and no one is accountable for the project plan.

Pitfalls of a team-driven plan can be avoided by taking control over the project and planning process. The nurse informatics specialist remains responsible for the project and facilitates the input from stakeholders and experts using group dynamics. The goal is to achieve consensus on issues related to the plan such as workflow, regulatory requirements, and policies and procedures. The final plan is developed by and coordinated by the nurse informatics specialist.

Project Sponsor and Steering Committees

The project sponsor has a key role in planning and throughout the life of the project. The project sponsor is the person within the healthcare facility who proposes the project to the administration and receives authorization to undertake the project. A project should not be started unless a person is clearly designated as the project sponsor.

The nurse informatics specialist should build relationship capital with the project sponsor immediately at the beginning of the project. The relationship should be trusting, and the project sponsor should be proactive and become an active participant in the project when necessary. At times the project sponsor will need to make critical decisions related to the project quickly (see SBAR). At other times the project sponsor will need to intervene in conflicts among stakeholders to keep the project on track. Some nurse informatics specialists refer to this as the Captain Kirk (*Star Trek*) project sponsor. Captain Kirk was noted for beaming down to personally resolve difficult issues on a planet.

In addition to the project sponsor, the nurse informatics specialist needs a **steering committee** assigned to the project by the project sponsor. The steering committee is composed of influential leaders within the healthcare facility who know policies and procedures and workflows from both a theoretic and pragmatic position. Typically, steering committee members are middle managers and other recognized leaders within the organization. Collectively, they have the experience to either directly respond to issues or know the right parties who can respond to issues.

The steering committee is the sounding board for the nurse informatics specialist who can present issues and proposed solutions to them so the steering committee can assess the importance of the issues and practicality of the solutions. Furthermore, the steering committee monitors key project metrics to determine if the project is on track.

Real-Time Planning

Real-time planning is a technique for modifying plans based on the current situation. General Norman Schwarzkopf championed real-time planning during Desert Storm when he said, "Timing is everything in battle, and unless we adjust the plan, we stand to lose momentum." The same situation exists with projects.

In traditional project management, the nurse informatics project manager is expected to predict future needs with certainty and then develop a schedule that meets those needs. The reality is that everything related to a project can be predicted with certainty, and therefore the plan, no matter how well thought out, will flounder when unexpected events occur.

The issue is how to respond to unexpected events because the plan does not address these situations. There is typically a hierarchy in a complex project, a chain of command that can extend to the COO of the healthcare facility, although it usually ends with the project sponsor. General Schwarzkopf determined that the higher in the chain of command, the less knowledgeable a person is about the unexpected event and therefore the less reliable the person's input into the decision on how to address the issue.

For example, a computer network specialist determines that the router (see Chapter 7) is inefficient and cannot adequately handle the new network traffic expected when the electronic medical record system goes live throughout the healthcare facility. Based on anticipated traffic flow provided by the vendor, another model router needs to be ordered and installed on the network. This is an unexpected event that can be addressed by the computer network specialist ordering a new router. Should this change in the plan be raised up the chain of command and approved by the project sponsor and the steering committee?

Traditional project management methodology requires that the change management process (see Chapter 5) be initiated. The change management process requires a detailed analysis of the issue and each option. The assessment is presented to the change management committee, which is likely to be the steering committee, which will evaluate the assessment and determine if the change should be implemented. If so, then the nurse informatics project manager modifies the project plan to reflect the change.

General Schwarzkopf questioned the value of the chain of command being involved in every unexpected event and solutions to address the event. The change management process, in this example, delayed addressing the event and therefore might have delayed the project. Furthermore, the remoteness of the change management committee to the event meant that they did not add any value to the decision. Their involvement did not change and would not change the decision.

NURSING ALERT

The change management process is a critical process to evaluate functionalities that were not part of the original project specifications. However, the project team should have authority to change the original project plan to address unexpected events that occur during development of the project.

Real-time planning requires meetings among the nurse informatics project manager, the project team, and relevant stakeholders to review current events. The meeting is short and direct and focuses on the managerial issues related to the changed event. For example, the meeting focuses on the expense, legal issues, timing issues, and vendor negotiations related to the new router—not technical issues.

Rapid Planning

Rapid planning occurs when little is predictable about the project. That is, the healthcare facility is embarking on uncharted waters. Initially, the project team and appropriate stakeholders gather to review the expectation for the project. Collectively, a decision is made as to the first task of the project plan. The task is performed, and the result of the task is reviewed. If the task is successful, then the next logical task is added to the plan, and that task is performed. If the task is unsuccessful, the gathering decides on a different direction (i.e., task). This concept is referred to as planning, deplanning, and replanning.

This is similar to how we find our way to a new destination (before GPS). Let's say there are three roads. We pick one and drive down the road looking for indications that we are on the right road (planning). After a mile or so, we determine this isn't the right road, and then we backtrack (deplanning) to the starting point. We then pick another road (replanning).

The **OODA loop model** is used to support rapid planning (Figure 6–1) by defining four stages in the decision process. These are:

- Observe: The initial step is to gather current information from as many sources that are available within the short time frame needed to make the decision.

- Orient: Analyze the information to determine if the information changes your current sense of reality related to the situation.

- Decide: Determine the next action that needs to be taken.

- Act: Act on your decision.

The action will provide feedback and then return to the beginning of the loop. This is the same process that you use when you are traveling in new surroundings.

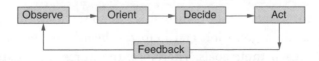

FIGURE 6–1 • The OODA (observe, orient, decide, act) loop is a model used to support rapid planning.

You move forward and gather new information that is assessed before determining if you are moving in the right direction. You decide to move forward or in a different direction and then do so and begin your decision-making process again.

Characteristics of Good Leadership

Administrators, stakeholders, the project sponsor, and the project team all look to the nurse informatics specialist to lead them through the complexity of developing and implementing a healthcare informatics system. There are characteristics that successful leaders exhibit and use to lead a diverse team through a complex maze of challenges that are posed by clinical information projects. These are:

- Commitment: The nurse informatics specialist needs to take ownership of the project and ensure that each participant has a stake in the success or failure of the project. Some project managers have referred to this as "having skin in the game." That is, each participant will experience the thrill of victory or the agony of defeat, as neatly said by ABC's Wide World of Sports. No participant can be absolved of responsibility.

- Change is your friend: Participants should be willing to start over at any time and junk plans that appear not to work. Furthermore, the project itself may be junked if the project is no longer viable for the healthcare facility. There is no sense continuing to follow a plan that does not produce results simply because time, money, and resources have already been invested in the plan.

- Quick success and quick failure: Identify when something is going right or wrong quickly so the plan can be adjusted accordingly. The sooner you know something doesn't work, the sooner you can redirect activities to something that might work.

- Celebrate failure: Knowing what doesn't work is as important as knowing what does work. The nurse informatics specialist should celebrate when a team member discovers that something does work because others on the team will know not to do it. Keeping failure a secret might result in others making the same mistake.

- People want to make a difference: It is safe to say that most people come to work to do a good job and help the healthcare organization—and patients—reach their goals. Therefore, the nurse informatics specialist must make all participants believe they are contributing.

- Give participants a sense of purpose: The nurse informatics specialist needs to clearly demonstrate how each participant's effort contributes to the overall project. This helps participants believe they are on a mission and not simply working on a project. Make sure that everyone clearly knows the purpose of the project.

- Participants support what they create: The nurse informatics specialist should assign each participant a task—a problem to solve—and let the participant determine how to solve the problem. Each participant has a sense of accomplishment and is quick to defend the entire project. Break down barriers that prevent participants from doing their jobs. Set guidelines within which tasks are to be performed and then hold the participants accountable for completing the tasks.

- Simplicity brings success: Express problems in simple terms so all participants can understand the problem regardless of their background. Likewise, ask participants to explain solutions in simple terms and consider simple solutions to the problem.

- Can-do attitude: Henry Ford reportedly said, "If you think you can, you can. If you think you can't, you can't. In either case you are right." The nurse informatics specialists must adopt a can-do attitude and install a can-do attitude in all participants.

- Keep lines of communication open: Formally and informally engage stakeholders in issues that are facing the project team so they can provide ongoing feedback that is likely to change the size of the program. Sharing the problem usually reduces the size of the problem because others may have options you didn't think of.

- Balanced life: There is more to life than the project. Encourage participants to strike an amiable balance between their personal life and working on the project. Likewise, the nurse informatics specialist must respect this balance.

- Open communication: Encourage all participants to voice any opinion without fear of reprisal. Each participant should have the courage to do the right thing. Everything should be out in the open with clearly defined tasks and who is responsible for each task.

CASE STUDY

CASE 1

Several weeks into the project to implement an electronic medical records application for the healthcare facility, the chief operating officer (COO) is concerned because he has not been informed of details relating to the progress on the project. Furthermore, he is concerned that the executive nurse hasn't been kept abreast of all details either. The COO asks you the following questions. What are your best responses?

QUESTION 1. Why do you allow members of the project team to make decisions without consulting you or the executive nurse?
ANSWER: Each member of the project team is a subject matter expert who is well informed of the goals of the project. Each team member is authorized to examine alternative solutions to problems affecting the task that she is working on and make an appropriate decision and implement that decision. No one on the project team or within the healthcare facility is more an expert than the team member; therefore, we are not in a position to reach a different decision. Time spent confirming the team member's decision delays implementation of that decision. Each team member knows when it is appropriate to raise the issue to a higher level in the chain of command.

QUESTION 2. Why do you use rapid planning techniques for some aspects of the project?
ANSWER: Aspects of the project that are predictable are included in the formal project plan; however, there are other aspects that no one can predict. In those situations, we use rapid planning. Rapid planning enables us to embark on an initial heading and then stop and evaluate whether or not that heading is correct. If we are going in the wrong direction, we take a step back, reevaluate options, and then choose a different heading.

QUESTION 3. Why should we trust your decisions?
ANSWER: Over the years, projects have been delivered successfully under my management. All information about my projects is open to all to see, and I allow stakeholders to be proactive and participate in the program when appropriate. This project has met expectations during the initial stages. Based on my reputation and our ongoing successful relationship, you can be assured that I will keep you appropriately involved in the project.

QUESTION 4. Why do you keep changing members of the project team?
ANSWER: There is a core group of specialists who stay on the project team throughout the life of the project. However, there are tasks that require certain expertise that we lack on the team. Subject matter experts join the project team to work on those specific tasks. When those tasks are completed, they return to their previous assignments.

FINAL CHECK-UP

1. **What is the purpose of a RACI chart?**
   A. A RACI chart identifies responsibility, accountability, and who has to be consulted and informed about the project.
   B. A RACI chart describes when tasks are scheduled to be performed.
   C. A RACI chart identifies tasks that have a direct impact on the project deadline.
   D. A RACI chart identifies the organization chart of the project.

2. **Why is it important for a nurse informatics project manager to know about group dynamics?**
   A. Group dynamics is used by the nurse informatics project manager to interact with patients.
   B. Group dynamics principles assist the nurse informatics project manager in addressing the needs of the project sponsor.
   C. Group dynamics is a management tool that helps the nurse informatics project manager assign tasks to resources.
   D. Understanding group dynamics can help the nurse informatics project manager to keep the project team and stakeholders focused on the project.

3. **What is the goal of mediation?**
   A. Mediation is a process in which the mediator decides the disputed issue.
   B. Mediation is a process in which the mediator helps two sides find common ground.
   C. Mediation is the process of avoiding conflicts.
   D. Mediation is the process of making decisions.

4. **What is the purpose of SBAR?**
   A. SBAR is a framework for mobile communications with practitioners.
   B. SBAR is a framework for describing a critical situation.
   C. SBAR is used for practitioners to communicate with other practitioners.
   D. SBAR is a framework for communicating effectively so decisions can be made quickly.

5. **How can timing be a barrier to effective communication?**

   A. The person receiving the message may not be in the frame of mind to listen and understand the message.

   B. The person sending the message may not have sufficient time to convey the message.

   C. The person sending the message may not have time to tell the receiver what the receiver is expected to do with the information.

   D. The person receiving the message will always have sufficient time to understand the message.

6. **What are the stages of adoption?**

   A. The stages of adoption is a process for adopting a proposal.

   B. The stages of adoption is the process of hiring a member of the project team.

   C. The stages of adoption is the process of developing the project charter.

   D. The stages of adoption is the process the project sponsor uses to accept the product of the project.

7. **What is a virtual team?**

   A. A virtual team is a project team that communicates using video conferencing and email.

   B. A virtual team is a project team in which participants join the team to complete specific tasks and then leave the team when the tasks are completed.

   C. A virtual team is a project team in which participants remain on the team for the length of the project.

   D. A virtual project team is a group of participants who move as a unit through a series of projects.

8. **What is relationship capital?**

   A. Relationship capital is the influence the nurse informatics specialist has with the MIS department.

   B. Relationship capital is the influence the nurse informatics specialist has with the vendor.

   C. Relationship capital is the ability to influence the project sponsor.

   D. Relationship capital is the reputation the nurse informatics specialist has with others in the healthcare facility that is used to build trust during a project.

9. **What is the purpose of a steering committee?**

   A. A steering committee is a group of nurses who provide input to the project.

   B. A steering committee is a group of clinicians who are responsible for the project.

   C. A steering committee is a group of influential leaders who act as a sounding board for the nurse informatics specialist during the life of the project.

   D. A steering committee is a group of clinicians who oversee development of the project.

10. **Why should one celebrate failure?**
    A. Knowing what does not work is just as important as knowing what does work.
    B. Celebration encourages the team members to try harder next time.
    C. Celebration acknowledges that the team members attempted doing the correct thing.
    D. Celebration helps to maintain self-esteem.

CORRECT ANSWERS AND RATIONALES

1. A. The RACI chart identifies responsibility, accountability, and who has to be consulted and informed about the project.
2. D. Understanding of group dynamics can help the nurse informatics project manager keep the project team and stakeholders focused on the project.
3. B. Mediation is a process in which the mediator helps two sides find common ground.
4. D. SBAR is a framework for communicating effectively so decisions can be made quickly.
5. A. The person receiving the message may not be in the frame of mind to listen and understand the message.
6. A. The stages of adoption is a process for adopting a proposal.
7. B. A virtual team is a project team in which participants join the team to complete specific tasks and then leave the team when the tasks are completed.
8. D. Relationship capital is the reputation that the nurse informatics specialist has with others in the healthcare facility that is used to build trust during a project.
9. C. A steering committee is a group of influential leaders who act as a sounding board for the nurse informatics specialist during the life of the project.
10. A. Knowing what does not work is just as important as knowing what does work.

chapter *7*

Clinical Computer Networks

LEARNING OBJECTIVES

1. Encoding data
2. Open Systems Interconnection model
3. Network packets
4. Ethernet and networks
5. Routers
6. IP addresses
7. The Internet and intranet
8. Remote login
9. Email
10. Wi-Fi
11. Bluetooth
12. Cell phones

KEY TERMS

Analog	Network
American Standard Code for	Packet switching
Information Interchange (ASCII)	Packets
Bridge	Point of Presence
Carrier-sense multiple access	Post Office Server (POP3)
Collision detection CSMA/CD	Protocols
Configuration table	Router
Digital	Simple Mail Transfer Protocol (SMTP)
Electromagnetic spectrum	Switch
Frame	TCP/IP
Hypertext Transfer Protocol (HTTP)	Tier 1 carriers
Internet Mail Access Protocol server	Unicode
(IMAP)	Uniform Resource Locator (URL)
Local Area Network (LAN)	Wave
Media Access Control (MAC)	Wide Area Network (WAN)

Think for a moment. How is the progress note entered a patient's electronic medical record transmitted to the electronic medical record application database and then made available to practitioners throughout the healthcare facility—and possibly outside the healthcare facility? The answer is that the progress note and other patient information are transmitted electronically over a computer **network**.

A network is both a physical and wireless connection among computers much like roadways connect houses and communities together. Each computer has a unique address similar to the street address of a house. Patient information is placed into an electronic envelope addressed to the destination computer, and the envelope is placed on the networks traveling to the destination computer.

This simple description of a computer network helps to frame the complexity of networking that is presented in this chapter. It is important for the nurse informatics specialist to have a working understanding of how a computer network functions and how information is transmitted within seconds over the network.

1. Encoding Data

The fundamental question of how information is transmitted over a network is answered by reviewing how information is encoded, which was discussed in Chapter 1. Letters, numbers, and symbols found on the keyboard are assigned a number according to the **American Standard Code for Information Interchange (ASCII)**.

Because there are insufficient numbers available in ASCII code to accommodate symbols used in every language such as Asian languages that use ideographs, engineers developed **Unicode**. Unicode contains two distinct blocks of code. One is called Unicode-2 and the other Unicode-4. Unicode-2 uses a 16-bit (two bytes) number to represent symbols. This means 65,536 distinct symbols can be assigned a Unicode-2 value. Unicode-4 uses a 32-bit (four bytes) number, which can handle about a million symbols.

> **NURSING ALERT**
>
> The first 255 numbers of Unicode are the same as ASCII.

A number assigned to the keyboard can be represented in the base 10 numbering (digits 0–9) or any other base numbering system. The base 10 numbering system, called the decimal system, is what is used daily in clinical calculations. Computers use a base 2 numbering system (digits 0–1) called the binary system. Figure 7–1 shows the word SMITH represented both as decimal and binary values.

Binary values are of particular use because each binary digit can be represented by the state of a **switch**—off/on. By manipulating a set of switches, we can encode any character that appears on the keyboard plus special characters called control characters that tell when to start a new page among other things.

Wave Properties

Imagine a still body of water interrupted by dropping a stone in the water. The energy of the stone striking water molecules causes each water molecule to push its neighboring molecule, causing the formation of a **wave**. The wave continues until all water molecules stop pushing at which time the body of water is still again.

SMITH		
Decimal		Binary
S = 83	=	1011 0011
M = 77	=	1010 1101
I = 73	=	1010 1001
T = 84	=	1011 0100
H = 72	=	1010 1000

FIGURE 7–1 • The word SMITH can be encoded into decimal and binary values.

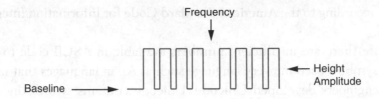

FIGURE 7–2 • A wave has properties. The baseline is where no wave action occurs. The amplitude is the height of the wave. The frequency is the number of waves per second.

A wave has certain properties. The still body of water is referred to the baseline at which point there is no wave. The height above the baseline of the wave is called the amplitude. The number of waves per second is called the frequency (Figure 7–2).

Notice that the height of the wave resembles the state of a switch. The baseline is as if the switch is off, and the height of the wave is as if the switch is on. Knowing this, we can encode a binary value in a wave just like the binary value is encoded in a set of switches. A 0 value is assigned to the baseline, and a 1 value is assigned to the height of the wave. Controlling when the wave is at baseline or at its height enables us to transmit 0s and 1s on a wave.

The Electromagnetic Spectrum

Waves are not only generated in water. Waves are also produced by moving any kind of molecule. For example, vibration of vocal cords sets air molecules moving, causing a wave to form. That wave has the same properties as the wave of water—amplitude and frequency.

The frequency of a wave determines the characteristic of the wave. For example, waves of a certain frequency can be heard by humans. Radio waves can travel 360 degrees and through some objects such as walls. Microwaves, commonly used in satellite television, travel in one direction and cannot go through objects. And lightwaves travel approximately 90 degrees and cannot go through most objects. All of these waves have the same properties. Therefore, information can be encoded into each of these waves.

The **electromagnetic spectrum** (Figure 7–3) groups waves into bands of frequencies, each band having similar characteristics.

Analog Waves and Digital Waves

An **analog** wave is generated by alternating electrical current causing the wave to fluctuate between above and below the baseline (Figure 7–4). The height of the wave above the baseline is called positive voltage. The height of the wave

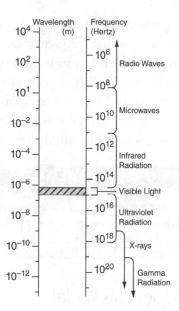

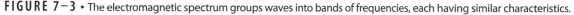

FIGURE 7−3 • The electromagnetic spectrum groups waves into bands of frequencies, each having similar characteristics.

below the baseline is called negative voltage. Negative voltage is assigned a 0 value, and positive voltage is assigned a 1 value. This enables encoding of information in an analog wave.

Until the introduction of **digital** technology, all communication was transmitted using analog waves because the waves can easily be generated using electricity and can be transmitted over long distances. Information was originally encoded into the amplitude of the analog wave. For example, waves generated by vocal cords cause a microphone element to vibrate. The microphone element was attached to an electromagnet that caused electrical current to fluctuate in synchronization with the voice. The electrical signal is then transmitted to the receiver, where the reverse process occurs. The current causes the electromagnet at the receiver to vibrate the element in the receiver that in turn vibrates air molecules and then our ears.

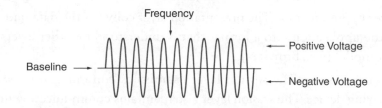

FIGURE 7−4 • An analog wave fluctuates between above and below the baseline.

An advantage of analog waves is that they can be transmitted over long distances. A drawback is waves of similar frequency can interfere with the transmitted wave, especially if the wave is transmitted through the air.

A digital wave (see Figure 7–1) consists of positive voltage. That is, the height of the wave is present (the value 1) or not present (the value 0). The form sometimes appears to have corners, which is why a digital wave is also called a square wave. Digital waves can be transmitted over short distances.

> **NURSING ALERT**
>
> Analog waves are still used to transmit signals; however, information is digitally encoded into the wave where positive voltage is the value 1 and negative voltage is the value 0. This process decreases the impact of signal interference.

2. Open Systems Interconnection Model

Information that is in a clinical application must be processed through several steps for the information to be transmitted over a network. These steps are called layers and are defined by the Open Systems Interconnection (OSI) model. The model was developed by the International Organization for Standardization and is widely used by nearly all networks.

There are seven layers in the OSI model. Each layer prepares the data for the next level. Layers are divided into two sets. These are the application set and the transport set. The application set focuses on preparing data from the application to be transported over the network and receiving preparing data that was received from the network. The transport set focuses on transporting the data.

The application set consists of three layers numbered from the highest to the lowest.

- Layer 7, application: The application layer prepares the data from the application to be transmitted over the network such as the person selecting the send button (MS Outlook).

- Layer 6, presentation: The presentation layer converts the data understood by the application into a format that is understood by other layers in the OSI model (e.g., browsers).

- Layer 5, session: The session layer establishes communication with the receiving device. The session layer also maintains communication until the message is received.

The transport set consists of four layers. These are:

- Layer 4, transport: The transport layer controls the flow of data and determines if there were any transmission errors. The transport layer also integrates data from multiple applications into a single stream of data.

- Layer 3, network: The network layer determines the way the data is sent over the network (i.e., IP address).

- Layer 2, data: The data layer defines the network type, packet sequencing and physical network **protocols** to use for the data (i.e., network card, MAC address).

- Layer 1, physical: The physical layer is the hardware that controls the timing of data, connections, and voltages (i.e., cables).

Protocols

A protocol is an agreed upon way of doing something. For example, we say hello when answering the telephone. This is a protocol for answering the telephone. When we call someone, we expect that person to answer with a hello. The same general concept is true with communicating over a network. That is, each layer of the OSI model is expected to receive data that is organized in a specific protocol. For example, **TCP/IP** is a term commonly used in networking. This refers to the transmission control protocol (TCP) and Internet protocol (IP). TCP/IP specifies the protocol for end-to-end connectivity over the Internet. This includes data formatting, addressing, transmission, routing, and how the information is received at the destination.

TCP/IP defines layers that correspond to some extent with the OSI model. These layers are referred to as a protocol stacks. Each protocol defines how a function is performed. The output of one protocol can be read as input to the next protocol.

- Layer 1, network interface: The network interface is a combination of the physical and data layers of the OSI model. This manages data exchange between the network and other devices.

- Layer 2, Internet: The Internet is similar to the network layer of the OSI model and determines the address of devices on the network.

- Layer 3, transport: Transport is similar to the transport layer of the OSI model because it is responsible for initiating communications with other network devices.

- Layer 4, application: Application is a combination of the application layer, presentation layer, and session layer in the OSI model and interfaces with applications that want to send or receive information from the network.

> **NURSING ALERT**
>
> The OSI model and the TCP/IP is the focus of developers who build software and hardware to deal with each layer. The nurse informatics specialist needs only to have an overview of the OSI model and TPC/IP.

3. Network Packets

Information that is transmitted over a network is broken down into relatively small pieces to form a packet. Think of a packet as an electronic envelop. Each packet maybe a fixed size measured in bytes. **Packets** are also known as a frame, block, cell, or segment depending on the type of network. A packet has three parts (Figure 7–5). These are:

- Header: The header contains information about the packet and includes the packet length, the network protocol, the destination address, the origination address, synchronization, and the packet number. The packet length is included because some networks have fixed or variable lengths. Network protocol is specified because some networks can use different types of protocols. Synchronization enables the packet to match the network. And the packet number is the number of the packets in the transmission.

- Body: The body is the pieces of the information that is contained in the packet. Sometimes the body also contains padding if the piece of information is less than the fixed length of the body of the packet.

- Trailer: The trailer contains information that identifies the end of the packet. The trailer may also contain error check information called the cyclic redundancy check (CRC). CRC is the sum of all binary ones. The receiving computer totals all the binary ones in the packet and compares them with the CRC value. If they match, then there is a likelihood that no error occurs. A mismatch indicates an error occurred, and a request is made to resend the packet.

Each packet is transmitted over the network passing through network devices such as a **router** that directs the packet through the maze of network connections toward its destination address. Think of a router as a post office. An envelope that you mail first arrives at the post office, where the envelope is read and

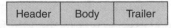

FIGURE 7–5 • A packet is similar to an envelope that has three parts. These are the header, body, and trailer.

forwarded to either the destination address or to a regional post office, where the envelope is further redirected until the envelop reaches its destination.

Packet numbers play an important role is transmitting information. Information is broken down into pieces and placed in a packet. Several packets may be needed to transmit the information. Each packet is given a number (e.g., packet 1 of 5). When the packet is received, software at the destination waits until all packets in the transmission are received, then packets are opened, and the information is reassembled and made available to the appropriate application.

> **NURSING ALERT**
>
> Moving packets around a network is called **packet switching**.

4. Ethernet and Networks

Now that you have a general idea of how a progress note is entered into the patient's electronic medical record is encoded into a format that is acceptable to a network, we will turn our attention to the network itself. A network enables computing devices to send and receive information from other computing devices.

There are two groups of network technologies. These are

- **Local Area Network (LAN)**: A LAN is a network technology that connects computing devices that are relatively close to each other such as in the same healthcare facility.

- **Wide Area Network (WAN)**: A WAN a is network technology that connects a smaller number of computing devices over a larger area such as connecting two or more healthcare facilities together.

> **NURSING ALERT**
>
> The term *computing devices* refers to any device on the network that can send and receive information. Although many of these devices are computers, some are devices that normally are not recognized as a computer such as a printer that is directly connected to the network.

The Beginnings of a Network

Ethernet is one of the most popular network technologies and was developed in 1973 by Bob Metcalfe at Xerox Corporation's Palo Alto Research Center. Metcalfe developed both the way to connect a cable to computers

(Ethernet connection) and the standards used to communicate over the connection to the other computing device.

Ethernet is used for LANs. Computing devices are connected to the Ethernet using a pathway that can transmit data. The pathway is better known as twisted pair cables, coaxial cable, or fiberoptic cable. These are referred to as the medium. Each computing device on the medium is referred to as a node, and the shared medium (cable) by two nodes is called an Ethernet segment commonly referred to as a segment. A group of pieces of information transmitted across the medium is referred to as a **frame**. A frame is another term used for a packet. A variable can be of variable size.

Based on the Ethernet protocol, each frame must have a destination address and a source address. Each address uniquely identifies a node on the Ethernet network. Furthermore, there are minimum and maximum lengths for frames.

The Flow Across the Ethernet

A frame sent by a source node is delivered to every node on the Ethernet network. Each node examines the frame and discards the frame if the destination address is not that of the node's address. Only the node with the matching destination address examines the content of the frame.

> **NURSING ALERT**
>
> The Ethernet protocol has a broadcast address. A broadcast address, commonly referred to as a broadcast, is assigned as the destination address of a frame if the computing device wants all nodes on the Ethernet network to examine the content of the frame. No node discards the frame, although each node can decide how to process the contents.

The Ethernet protocol requires that frames be regulated using **carrier-sense multiple access** with **collision detection (CSMA/CD)**. All nodes have equal access to send a frame across the Ethernet network. However, before a node transmits a frame, the node listens to the network to hear if another node is transmitting a frame. This is referred to as carrier sense. The node sends the frame if the network is clear of traffic.

However, there can be a time when two nodes decide to send a frame at the same time. Both listen to the network and determine there is no traffic on the network, so both send a frame. The two frames collide, commonly referred to as a collision. Each node that sends a frame receives the frame, too. The node assesses if the frame is intact. If so, then the node knows there was no collision. However, if the frame was garbled, then the node realizes that the frame collided with at least one other frame on the network.

When a collision is detected, the node stops sending the frame. After a random amount of time, the node resends the frame after determining that the network is clear of traffic. The random time to pause makes it unlikely that the other node that sent the colliding frame will resend the frame at the exact same time.

Limitations

One would think that all we need is to install a longer cable if more computing devices need to join the network. In reality, there are limitations to the Ethernet and to cables. The longer the distance the transmission travels, the weaker the signal becomes. Imagine the wave in a pond of water. The wave is strongest at the site when the stone is thrown into the pond. The wave diminishes greatly the farther the wave moves away from the site.

Interference is another limitation of the Ethernet network. Interference occurs when a different transmission source sends a signal that is similar to the signal transmitted on the Ethernet network, which causes both signals to become garbled. You might have experienced this using a hardwired telephone when you hear another conversation on the telephone during your conversation. This is called cross-talk and is a form of interference.

Besides distance and interference, Ethernet has another limitation—the number of computing devices that can exist on the same network. Remember that each device must wait until the network is clear of traffic before transmitting a frame. The more computing devices on the network, the higher the chance that multiple computing devices want to transmit frames at the same time, resulting in collisions of frames and transmission delays.

> **NURSING ALERT**
>
> These limitations are not only limitations of Ethernet but are also limitations found in other network technologies.

Solutions to Network Limitations

The signal along the network diminishes as the signal is transmitted along the network. Therefore, the signal is effective for a specific distance that is determined on the medium used for the network. For example, the signal over a coaxial cable medium is 500 meters (1640 feet). To extend the effective distance for the signal, engineers install a repeater. A repeater is a device that receives the signal and then retransmits the signal. Think of this like someone telling you a message, and then you pass that message along to the next person. Although the message is the same, you are using your own voice to generate the sound wave. You are simply repeating the message. A repeater can connect multiple segments of the network similar to your relaying the message to several people.

Congestion on the network is an increasing problem as more computing devices join the network. There is a high likelihood that multiple computing devices will want to transmit at the same time. The congestion problem is addressed by dividing the network into smaller networks, each called a segment. Each segment has a manageable number computing devices, avoiding potential transmission delays. Think of this as breaking up a big city into several smaller cities that are relatively easier to manage.

Bridge and Router

Dividing the network into segments presents a new problem. Computing devices on one segment are unable to communicate with computing devices on a different segment because no connection exists between segments. Engineers addressed this problem by creating a **bridge**. A bridge is an electronic device that regenerates the signal similar to the actions of a repeater and regulates network traffic, enabling frames to be exchanged among segments. The bridge reduces unnecessary network traffic by examining the destination address of each frame. If the destination address is for a computing device on the other segment, then the bridge forwards the frame to the segment, enabling the destination computing device to receive the frame. However, a frame having a destination address of a computing device on a different segment is dropped by the bridge. That is, the frame is not forwarded to the other segment because the bridge knows that segment does not have the destination address.

A problem with a bridge is that segments are physical connections to the bridge; another problem is that Ethernet broadcasts are sent to all segments connected to the bridge. Remember that an Ethernet broadcast is received by every computing device on the network. As additional computing devices join the network and additional bridges connect multiple segments, traffic congestion can develop.

A router replaces the bridge to alleviate congestion. A router is an electronic device that logically divides a network (see Routers) into segments. Furthermore, a router uses rules (protocols) that are different than Ethernet. This means that a router can connect a variety of network technologies.

Switches

Switched Ethernet changes the image of a segment. In a switched Ethernet, there is one computing device on a segment rather than multiple computing devices on a segment. No longer do computing devices share the same medium.

This means that some segments can use fiberoptics and others coaxial cable, and still others twist pair wires, depending on the technological requirements for the computing device. A computing device connects to the medium, and the medium is connected to the switch. A switch can handle hundreds of segments.

A frame is sent from the sending computing device to the switch. The switch reads the destination address on the frame and then forwards the frame only to the segment that contains the destination address. A primary benefit of a switch is the reduction of traffic across segments. That is, the frame travels from the sender's segment to the switch and to the receiver's segment. No other segments receive the frame. In addition, multiple computing devices can transmit a frame simultaneously because the switch manages the network traffic flow. There are no collisions. Switches also enable computing devices to transmit and receive frames at the same time. This is referred to as full duplex.

NURSING ALERT

There are technologies other than Ethernet. These include IBM's token ring, where a packet called a token is passed among computing devices on the network. A computing device needs the token to transmit data. Asynchronous transfer mode (ATM) is another network technology that can transmit video, voice, and data at high speeds over long distances.

---

5. Routers

A router is a networking device that can join together two network segments that use the same or different technology and sees every packet that is transmitted. When the router receives a packet, the router looks at the destination address in the packet and then forwards the packet to the destination, similar to your local post office sorting and redirecting mail. Figure 7–6 shows a very simple network where nodes are connected to a router. A second router connects other routers to small networks and the backbone network. Think of a backbone network as a superhighway that leads to servers, mainframes, and other high-demand computing devices.

The router uses a **configuration table**, sometimes referred to as a router table, to determine where to forward a packet. The configuration table has the network connection that leads to a group of destination addresses. Many times the connection is to another router, which performs the same task. This sequence continues until a router locates the actual destination address.

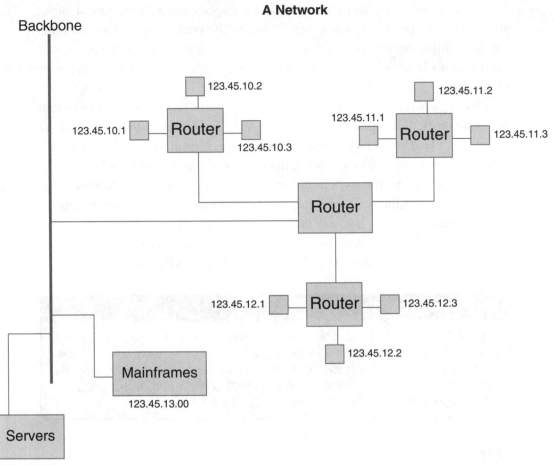

A Network

Backbone

123.45.10.2

123.45.10.1 — Router

123.45.10.3

123.45.11.2

123.45.11.1

Router — 123.45.11.3

Router

123.45.12.1 — Router — 123.45.12.3

123.45.12.2

Mainframes

123.45.13.00

Servers

123.45.14.00

FIGURE 7–6 • A simple network diagram in which computing devices are connected to routers and a router connects together other routers, enabling packets to cross over networks.

The configuration table can be a few lines for routers on relatively small networks or extremely large for routers that handle massive amounts of traffic such as traffic on the Internet.

At first this may sound confusing, but it will be clear if you think of a router as the post office. The postal carrier picks up mail at your mailbox or a mailbox on the street and brings the mail to the post office (router). The destination address has a postal code. The postal worker (or machine) examines the postal code to determine if the destination address is in the same community as the post office. If so, then the mail is placed in a slot designated for the destination address, and the next day the post carrier delivers the mail to the destination. This is the connection that leads to the destination address.

However, the postal code may be for a different community. The mail is then placed in a pouch destined for a regional post office (router). There the mail is sorted and placed in the pouch going to the post office that serves the destination address (router). This process continues until the mail is delivered to the destination address.

The configuration table has priorities of connection. That is, the router sends the packet to the router that is closest to the destination address. However, there can be occasions when either the network connects to the router or the router itself is not working. The router then sends the packet to the second closest router to the destination address. That is, the packet is redirected around a traffic jam.

Another piece of information in the configuration table includes rules for routing packets and rules for handling special traffic.

As the number of networks joins to form larger interconnected networks, network traffic also increases. Through the use of the configuration table, the router or routers are able to deliver packets efficiently while reducing congestion on the network by redirecting packets only to connections that lead to the destination address. A router can find the most direct connection to the destination address regardless of the size and complexity of the joined networks.

> **NURSING ALERT**
>
> You can track to number of routers used to reach a destination by using tracert. Open the command prompt window in Windows, enter tracert www.google.com, and then press the enter key. The number of routers used to reach Google will be displayed along with their IP addresses.

Packet Switching

The path traveled by a packet from the originating computing device to the destination computing device may involve many different networks, especially if transmission occurs over the Internet. The Internet is a network operating mostly by major telephone companies referred to as **Tier 1 carriers**.

Tier 1 carriers create a circuit between two points on the network using an assortment of routers and mediums. A circuit is a connection. It is common for a circuit to begin with a coaxial connection from the healthcare facility to a fiberoptic connection that carries the packet to the Tier 1 carrier's switcher. From there, the packet may travel to and from a satellite using microwaves to a Tier 1 carrier's receiving station and then over a fiberoptic connection to the coaxial cable that leads into the destination facility.

The Tier 1 carrier's network is commonly referred to as a packet-switching network because the primary purpose of the network is to use routers to redirect packets. Packets on a Tier 1 carrier's network are relatively large at roughly 1500 bytes.

A packet-switching network is designed with redundancy and use a technique called load balancing to ensure packets reach their destinations within an acceptable time period, typically measured in milliseconds. If a delay is detected due to equipment malfunction, the packet-switching network automatically reroutes the packet to a different circuit.

> **NURSING ALERT**
>
> Packet-switching networks are used for telephone calls. The caller's voice is digitized and divided into packets.

Routers come with different capabilities. Some routers are designed for a home network, but others can handle the needs of a healthcare facility. More robust routers handle massive amounts of traffic and are capable of reconfiguring the configuration table based on traffic flowing over the network. For example, the router monitors the time necessary to deliver packets to a destination address that is a member of a group of addresses (same postal code). The router has the capability to create a different route if a delay is encountered on the connection to the destination address. This can happen if there is equipment failure somewhere along the connection in the massive network.

Each router needed to make the connection between the originating address and the destination address is commonly called a hop. That is, the packet hops from router to router on its way to the destination address. Each hop causes a millisecond delay. The more hops, the more delay. In a robust network, the delays are not noticed because there are many alternative connections (i.e., routers) available. On less robust networks, the delay may be noticed, and users of the network will report decreased response times. Response time is the lapse of time between an action such as sending and receiving a request of the network.

Network Addresses

A router needs to know the destination address and the network of the destination computing device. The destination computing device has two addresses. There are the physical address of the computing device and the logical address. The physical address is called the **Media Access Control (MAC)** address that is permanently stored on the computing device's network interface card (NIC). The MAC address is 6 bytes. The first 3 bytes identify the manufacturer of the NIC, and the last 3 bytes is the NIC series number. The combination makes the MAC unique.

The logical address is the address of the computing device on the network, which depends on the type of network in use. The most commonly used logical address is the IP address. The originating computing device uses a logical address to send a packet to a destination computing device over the network.

The format of the logical address is determined by the network protocol such as TCP/IP for the Internet. There are many different networks, each having a network protocol. The router is designed to interact with the most common networks, enabling computing devices to communicate to other computing devices on different networks. The router can translate a packet from one network protocol to a different network protocol.

6. IP Addresses

An IP address is either a static address or a dynamic address. A static address is a fixed IP address for the computing device that does not change. However, many computing devices use dynamic IP addresses that are assigned by a program on the network using the Dynamic Host Configuration Protocol (DHCP). Each time the computing device connects to the network, the DHCP service assigns the computing device an IP address that is used until the computing device disconnects from the network.

An IP address is divided into four 8-digit binary numbers. Each can be a number from 0 to 255. Some numbers are reserved by the Internet Assigned Numbers Authority (IANA) for special network functions. Reserved IP addresses are:

- 0.0.0.0: Default network.
- 255.255.255.255: Network broadcast. All computing devices receive packets with this destination address.
- 127.0.0.1: Called loopback addresses and used by a computing device to identify itself.
- 169.254.0.1 to 169.254.255.254: Called the Automatic Private IP Addressing (APIPA) range. An IP address within this range is automatically assigned if the computing device is not assigned a dynamic IP address by the DHCP.

> **NURSING ALERT**
>
> The Internet is running out of IP addresses. Currently, IP addresses are version IPv4 and consist of a 32-bit address system that can support 4,294,967,296 unique IP addresses. That is, an IP address has 32 bits. The Internet Engineering Task Force (IETF) was formed in the early 1990s to create a new version called IPv6 that consists of a 128-bit address system in which each IP address has 128 bits.

Subnet

A subnet is a segment of a large network. All subnets are connected by a router. Each subnet is usually assigned an IP address. The router uses the assigned IP address to know which subnet to send a destination packet. Subnet addresses are grouped into classes identified by letters that are reserved for subnets. Classes A, B, and C rangers are commonly assigned to a subnet. Classes D and E IP addresses are used for special purposes.

A block of IP addresses is assigned by the IANA to businesses and government agencies. Each then reassigns IP addresses to computing devices and subnets within their organization. Most consumers connect to the Internet through an Internet Service Provider (ISP). An ISP is a business that is assigned a block of IP addresses. The ISP temporarily assigns one of those IP addresses to the consumer when the consumer's computing device connects to the ISP service.

Many consumers have a router. Computing devices are either connected to the router using a cable or through a wireless connection. This forms a home network. Each computing device on the home network is on a subnet and has its own IP address. That IP address identifies the computing device on the home network. Each computing device connects to the Internet through the router. The dynamic IP address assigned by the ISP is assigned to the router. The router receives packets from computing device on the home network and forwards those packets to the ISP. Likewise, packets received by the router are forwarded to the appropriate computing device on the home network.

A subnet IP address has two parts. One part identifies the subnet and the other part identifies the computing device (node) on the subnet. The node is also referred to as the host. The size of each part is measured in bits depending on the number of subnets and the number of nodes. A network that has many subnets, each having a relatively few computing devices on each subnet, will reserve 24 bits of the subnet's IP address for the subnet and 8 bits for each node. Conversely, a network with few subnets and many computing devices on each subnet will reserve 8 bits of the IP address to identify the subnet and 24 bits to identify each node. The network administrator can adjust the size of the parts of the subnet IP address based on the need of the network.

NURSING ALERT

An IP address is divided into four sections (255.255.255.255). Each section has 8 bits (combinations of 0s and 1s). Parts of the subnet IP address are created by grouping the first, second, and/or third sections to identify the subnet. The fourth section is always used to identify the node on the subnet.

A subnet mask is used by computing devices to separate the subnet IP address. A series of 1 bits masks the portion of the IP address that identifies the subnet. A series of 0 bits masks the node portion of the IP address. Subnet masks are usually represented in decimal values rather than binary values. In decimal 0 (zero) is the same as 00000000 in binary. Likewise, 255 in decimal is the same as 11111111.

A subnet mask for a network that has few subnets with each subnet having many computing devices that will look like 255.0.0.0. In contrast, a network that has many subnets, each having a relatively few computing devices will have a subnet mask that looks like 255.255.255.0.

NURSING ALERT

Each section of an IP address can represent a maximum of 256 (decimal). That means a subnet with a subnet mask of 255.255.255.0 can have no more than 256 computing devices on the subnet. However, the network can have a maximum of 16,777,216 subnets. Keep in mind that some IP addresses are reserved, so the actual number might be less.

---

7. The Internet and Intranet

The Internet is a global network of networks connected by powerful routers operated by telecommunication companies using the TCP/IP protocols. No one owns the Internet. The Internet Society oversees protocols and policies for using the Internet. Telecommunication companies have a backbone network divided into regions. Each region has a **Point of Presence (POP)** where the network can be accessed such as an ISP. This is referred to as a Network Access Point (NAP). Each backbone (i.e., telecommunication company) connects to other backbones (other telecommunication companies), enabling transmission of packets over the Internet to any NAP throughout the world.

An intranet works on the same basic principles of the Internet except that an intranet is a private network typically within an organization. The World Wide Web (WWW) is a way to share information over the Internet using the **Hypertext Transfer Protocol (HTTP)**.

A computing device can access information over the Internet in one of two ways. First, the computing devices can use the File Transfer Protocol (FTP) to request a file from another computing device on the network, which is usually a server. A server is a computing device that has a special function such as serving web pages, serving applications, or serving files. FTP requests are written in a file and sent across the Internet or the request can be interactively made using a command prompt; on Windows, computers can be found in the accessories folder.

Uniform Resource Locator

The most common way to access information over the Internet is by using a browser. A browser is an application that enables someone to enter either a website name or the IP address of the server that hosts the website. It is common to use the website name rather than the IP address. The website name is called the **Uniform Resource Locator (URL)** and begins with www followed by a unique name and extension such as www.jimkeogh.com. The www is the name of the web server that hosts the website. The extension, such as .com, .edu, and .gov, is referred to as a top-level domain. The website name must be unique within the top-level domain. That is, there can be only one jimkeogh.com.

A request is made usually by the ISP to a domain name server (DNS) to translate the website name to the IP address of the server that hosts the website. Many DNS are available on the Internet. Each has a list of website names and the corresponding IP address.

Sometimes the ISP has its own DNS to reduce the time to retrieve the IP address. The DNS provides the IP address that corresponds to the URL or contacts another DNS server for the IP address. The DNS may simply send a return message saying that the URL is not known. Alternatively, the DNS can say the URL is unknown and provide the IP address of another DNS.

Web Server

A web server is a computing device that stores websites and files associated with the website such as videos and pictures. Each web server is assigned a unique IP address. Furthermore, a web server is connected to the network (i.e., Internet) through one or more communications ports commonly referred to as a port. Each port is identified by a number and supports a specific type of communication.

When a request is sent to the web server, the request contains the IP address of the web server and the port number. Port 21 is used for FTP requests, and port 80 is used for website request. When connected to the port, the web server interacts with the transmission using the corresponding protocol. That is, the file transfer protocol is for an FTP request, and the HTTP is for website requests.

In the FTP request, the web server authenticates the right to access the specified file, and if access is granted, a copy of the file is sent using the same port to the originator of the request.

In the HTTP request, the web server sends a copy of index.html to the originator of the request. This is commonly referred to as the home page for the website. The content of the file is written in hypertext markup language (HTML). HTML tells the browser how to display the page. The file typically has highlighted words called a hyperlink that when selected causes the browser to make another request to the web server for another page of the website.

8. Remote Login

A remove login enables a computing device called a host to take control over a remote computing device that is connected to the network. Both computers must be running the desktop sharing software. The remote computing device must give permission to the host computing device to access the computing device. Furthermore, the host computing device must also be running a viewer program that displays the screen of the remote computing device on the screen of the host computing device. All keystrokes, mouse clicks, and other input at the host computing device related to the display of the remote computing device is sent over the network to the remote computing device. The remote computing device treats the input as if the input was done using its input devices. Everything displayed on the remote computing device is also sent to the host computing device and is typically displayed in a window on the host computing device.

Telenet

Telenet is a software available to most computing devices that is used for remote logins. Telenet is available on most computing devices at the command prompt. The name telenet followed by the IP address of the remote computing device is entered at the command line. When the host successfully logs in, the command prompt on the host screen is the command prompt on the remote computing device.

> ### NURSING ALERT
>
> Windows computing devices may have telnet turned off. Telenet can be activated by going to the Control Panel and then Programs and then selecting Turn Windows Features On or Off. Select telenet client. Go to the command prompt and enter telenet.

Technology that enables remote login has been embellished to provide remote customer support, collaboration on projects, remote training classes, and the ability to share applications.

9. Email

Email is one of the most used applications on the Internet and intranet. An email message consists of short pieces of text, and sometimes longer files are attached to the message. The message is written into an email application called an email client. The email client also displays incoming emails and is used to manage emails. There are many kinds of email clients such as Microsoft Outlook that usually come with the computing device's operating system or are provided by the organization that provides the email service such as Google or Yahoo!

There are two email servers. These are the **Simple Mail Transfer Protocol (SMTP)** server and the **Post Office Server (POP3)**. The SMTP server sends emails, and the POP3 server receives emails. Another type of email server called the **Internet Mail Access Protocol server (IMAP)** handles both incoming and outgoing emails.

Each email server has an IP address and a port connection that connects the server to the network. The SMTP server uses port 25, POP3 uses port 110, and IMAP uses port 143.

SMTP

The email client sends the email to the SMTP server. The email will have a destination address such as myname@myserver.com. The SMTP receives the email from port 25 and then decomposes the destination address into two parts.

TABLE 7–1 A Sample of SMTP Commands

Command	Description
HELO	Introduction
EHLO	Introduction and requesting extended mode
MAIL FROM	Sender address
RCPT TO	Destination address
DATA	The first three lines are TO, FROM, and Subject followed by the body of the email message
RSET	Reset
QUIT	End session

These are the name of the person receiving the email (myname) and the domain name (myserver.com). The SMTP server uses the DNS to retrieve the IP address of the domain myserver.com. The SMTP server then sends the email to the web server that is associated with the corresponding IP address. The web server reads the destination address and places the email into the person's email box.

If the SMTP server is unable to connect to the IP address, the email is placed in the sendmail queue. Every 15 minutes for 4 hours, the SMTP server will try to resend the email. If the email still isn't delivered, the email client receives notice of the delay; after 5 days, the email is returned to the email client as undeliverable.

The email client reformats the email message into a format that is understood by the SMTP server. The format includes text commands to tell the SMTP what to do. Table 7–1 contains a sample of these commands.

POP3

The email client connects to the POP3 server to retrieve emails for a specific account. The request provides the user ID and password. After the login is authenticated, the email client requests that emails be transmitted to the email client. Table 7–2 contains a sample of POP3 commands. Typically, the email client will request a list of emails in the user's email account and display the list on the screen. When the user selects an email to open, another request is made by the email client to the POP3 server to retrieve that specific email. The email client can also request the first several lines of the email to preview the content on the screen. Also, the user can select an email to be deleted from the user's email account.

TABLE 7–2 A Sample of POP3 Commands

Command	Description
USER	User ID
USER	Password
QUIT	End session
LIST	Retrieve a list of emails and their size
RETR	Retrieve a specific email based on the position of the email on the list of emails
DELE	Delete a specific email based on the position of the email on the list of emails
TOP	Retrieve the first X lines of a specific email

NURSING ALERT

POP3 servers do not retain an email that was downloaded to the email client. After it is downloaded, the email is not available to another email client. That is, you are unable to read the same emails on two computing devices.

IMAP

The IMAP server enables users to organize emails into folders. Those folders appear in the client and on the IMAP server, enabling the email to be read by another client. Searching for an email occurs on the IMAP server and not on the email client. A drawback to using IMAP is that the email client must be connected to the IMAP server to read emails unless the email client copies all emails to the local computing devices. This process is called a cache and enables the email client to access emails even when the computing device is not connected to the network.

NURSING ALERT

Telenet can be used to send and request email without using an email client. Connection is made to the email server's IP address and to the port of the email server. The SMTP server uses port 25, and the POP3 uses port 110. IMAP uses port 143. Next send the proper commands to the email server. In essence, this is what the email client is doing.

Attachment

An email attachment is a long file that is to be sent along with the body of the email. This might be a photograph, word processing document, or practically any kind of file. However, the email client may set limitations such as file size restricting files that can be attached to an email.

Although the attachment appears as a line on the screen in the email client, the attachment remains as a separate file. The email client sends the email server a command that tells the email server that there is an attachment and then sends the attachment file to the email server followed by the email. The email server then places the email in the destination account. The email has reference to the attachment.

When the email client requests a list of emails, the email client is notified if the email has an attachment. After the email is opened, the user can request the email client to open the attachment. The email client then contacts the email server and retrieves the attachment file and displays the file on the screen.

10. Wi-Fi

Wi-Fi is a wireless network that uses radio waves to connect a computing device to the network. Circuits in the computing device digitally encode an analog radio wave and transmit the wave using an antenna to a router that also uses an antenna to receive the signal (see Encoding Data). When the signal is received, the digital data is decoded and sent to the destination computing device by the router. The router is commonly referred to as a wireless router, although the router is connected to the network using an Ethernet connection (see Ethernet and Networks).

Wi-Fi transmissions are either at 2.4 Ghz or 5 Ghz. One Ghz is 1 billion cycles (waves) per second. This is a higher frequency than cell phone (see Cell Phones). Wi-Fi uses the 802.11 network protocol. Some Wi-Fi computing devices transmit on one frequency or rapidly transmit on different frequencies referred to as frequency hopping. Frequency hopping reduces interference and enables the frequency to be shared.

An area that is accessible to the wireless network is called a Wi-Fi hotspot. Wi-Fi hotspots are provided by businesses, governments, and educational institutions, and consumers can create a hotspot using a mobile device with a cell phone. Wireless routers used at home are also hotspots. Many Wi-Fi hotspots cover an area of approximately 100 feet, however, electronic devices can be added to the network to extend the range.

Wireless routers require computing devices to log into the wireless router; otherwise, any computing device within a hotspot area can access the wireless network. See Chapter 10 to learn how to secure a Wi-Fi network.

> ### NURSING ALERT
>
> Wireless signals may become disrupted by the environment, including inside the healthcare facility. Therefore, technicians need to assess whether or not areas of the healthcare facility can access the wireless network.

11. Bluetooth

Bluetooth is a protocol that enables computing devices and electronic devices to connect with each other using a low-powered radiofrequency transmitter transmitting at 2.45 Ghz. The signal is weak, requiring the sending and receiving devices to be near each other, within a 32-foot radius. The weak signal also reduces the likelihood that other devices will interfere with the Bluetooth signal. Bluetooth is transmitted using frequency hopping, changing frequencies 1600 times per second to further avoid interference. Up to eight devices can be connected using Bluetooth.

When two Bluetooth devices are within range of each other, both devices automatically begin to communicate with each other. The range of a Bluetooth device is called a personal-area network (PAN) and is also known as piconet.

12. Cell Phones

Cell phone technology is used for sending text, checking email, and interacting with clinical applications remotely as well as being used for phone calls. Cell phones use radio waves to transmit and receive data over the cell phone network. The cell phone network is connected to a telecommunication company's large network—the same network that connects most computing devices that are available on the Internet.

Geographical areas are divided into sections called cells. A cell is typically 10 square miles in a hexagonal grid. Each cell has a base station that receives and sends data to cell phone within the cell. Cell phones and computing devices that use cell phone technology have a low transmission range sufficient to reach the base station within the cell.

Each cell phone carrier has about 800 radiofrequencies that can be used by cell phones within a cell. Because the cell phone's transmission range is relatively small, the same frequencies can be used in all cells. Two frequencies are used per call—one to transmit and the other to receive data. This is referred to as a duplex channel. The channel consists of two frequencies. Some frequencies are reserved to transmit data that controls the cellular transmission itself. All base stations for a cell phone carrier are connected to the Mobile Telephone Switching Office (MTSO). The MTSO forwards data to and from the land-line telephone system.

> **NURSING ALERT**
>
> A benefit of a cell phone having a low transmission range is that less power is needed to transmit the signal, resulting in lower power consumption.

Transmission

The cell phone automatically monitors the control channel for a System Identification Code (SID) that is transmitted by the base station. A message saying that 'no service is available' is displayed by the cell phone if the cell phone does not receive a SID. A SID is also programmed into the cell phone by the cell phone carrier. The cell phone knows if the cell phone is connected to the carrier's network if both the SID on the control channel and the SID programmed in the cell phone are the same.

When connected, the cell phone sends the base a registration request. The base forwards the registration request to the MTSO so the MTSO knows which cell the cell phone is using so the user can receive incoming calls. The MTSO also sends over the control channel to the cell phone telling the cell phone which two frequencies to use for transmission. The cell phone then begins transmission. As the cell phone signal weakens, the base station hands off the cell phone's transmission to the base station of the neighboring cell, enabling transmission to continue seamlessly.

A process called roaming occurs if the SID programmed into the cell phone does not match the SID of the base station. The base station forwards the SID to the MTSO. The MTSO contacts the MTSO of the cell phone's carrier to confirm the SID. After confirmation, the base station's MTSO processes the transmission. Most cell phones display a message indicating that roaming has occurred.

> **NURSING ALERT**
>
> There are two other codes in the cell phone. These are the Mobile Identification Number (MIN) that identifies the phone based on the cell phone number and the Electronic Serial Number (ESN) that is entered by the cell phone manufacturer to identify the cell phone. The MIN and ESN uniquely identify the cell phone.

Generations

Cell phones are commonly identified by generation such as 3G and 4G. The number refers to the generation of the cell phone. First-generation (1G) cell phones used analog technology (see Analog Waves and Digital Waves). Second-generation (2G) cell phones used digital technology. Digital technology enables more channels (two frequencies) with the bandwidth of cellular technology. Bandwidth is the number of frequencies that can be transmitted over a medium at the same time. Think of a highway. Bandwidth is the number of lanes in the highway.

Third-generation (3G) cell phone technology is capable of transmitting multimedia because of increased bandwidth and transmission speed across the network. Fourth-generation (4G) cell phone technology has the capability of providing HD TV, teleconferencing, and other applications that were traditionally reserved for desktop computing devices.

CASE STUDY

CASE 1

The chief nursing officer is considering the expansion of the clinical automation program in the healthcare facility. She realizes that a robust network is necessary to support the program. Currently, the healthcare facility has an electronic medical records system. Over the next 2 years, the facility wants to include an electronic medication administration system, an order management system, and a computer practitioner order entry system. She plans to meet with the management information systems (MIS) department to discuss the healthcare facility's network and proposed network upgrades. Before the chief nursing officer meets with the MIS department, she has the following questions about the network. What are your best responses?

QUESTION 1. What is bandwidth?

ANSWER: Bandwidth is the number of frequencies that can be transmitted over the network. Think of the network as a network of highways. Each lane represents a frequency. The greater the number of lanes (i.e., frequency), the more traffic can cross the network at the same time. Bandwidth depends on the technology used to transmit over the network.

QUESTION 2. How can practitioners review patient records and write orders remotely?

ANSWER: Mobile computing devices such as cell phones, smartphones, and tablets use cell phone technology to remotely log into the healthcare facility's network. The mobile computing devices connect to the nearest base station in the cell. The base station connects to the Mobile Telephone Switching Office (MTSO), which transmits message between the mobile computing devices over the Tier 1 carrier's network to the hospital's network.

QUESTION 3. How can the healthcare facility's network be extended without incurring the cost of running new network cables?

ANSWER: Wi-Fi technology can be used to expand the reach of the healthcare facility's network with limited cost of running new cables. Wi-Fi uses radio waves to transmit information among computing devices and the network. MIS needs to install Wi-Fi hotspots throughout the healthcare facility. Each Wi-Fi hotspot must be connected to the network via a cable. However, computing devices that are Wi-Fi capable do not need a network cable connection. Instead, the computing devices will connect to the Wi-Fi hotspot using a radio transceiver to send and receive information over the network.

QUESTION 4. How are computing devices recognized on the network?

ANSWER: Each computing device has a network interface card, sometimes referred to as the network card. Each network card has a unique address called the Media Access Control (MAC). Furthermore, each computing device is assigned a logical address called an Internet Protocol (IP) address. Information transmitted over the network is addressed to the destination computing device's IP address. The IP address corresponds to the MAC number and therefore is able to be delivered to the destination computing device.

FINAL CHECK-UP

1. What code is used to encode characters on the keyboard so the characters can be transmitted over the network?

   A. Binary
   B. ASCII
   C. Decimal
   D. Hex

2. **How is digital information encoded on an analog wave?**

    A. A wave's peak is considered a binary 1, and a wave's trough is considered a binary 0.

    B. A wave's frequency determines the binary value.

    C. A wave's length determines the binary value.

    D. An analog wave cannot be encoded with digital data.

3. **What is a network packet?**

    A. Fiberoptic transmission.

    B. Email.

    C. An electronic envelop used to transmit frames over the network.

    D. An electronic envelop used to transmit information over the network.

4. **What is the purpose of CSMA/CD?**

    A. To detect network traffic and collisions of nodes.

    B. To detect network traffic and collisions of packets.

    C. To detect network traffic.

    D. To detect network traffic and collision of MAC on the network.

5. **How many network segments are connected by a router?**

    A. 2

    B. 256

    C. 255

    D. An endless number of segments

6. **What is a node?**

    A. A device connected to the network.

    B. A device connected directly to a router.

    C. A device connected directly to a switch.

    D. A device connected directly to bridge.

7. **What is packet switching?**

    A. The transfer of packets inside a computing device.

    B. The transfer of packets between networks.

    C. OSI model.

    D. A circuit in a fiberoptic network.

8. **What is the IP address 255.255.255.255?**

    A. APIPA

    B. Loopback address

    C. Default network

    D. Network broadcast

9. **What is the primary benefit of IMAP?**

   A. Emails remain on the email server.

   B. Emails remain on the local computer.

   C. Emails remain in cache.

   D. Emails cannot be deleted.

10. **What is a computing device?**

   A. Any device on a wireless network.

   B. Any device that can calculate.

   C. Any device that can interact with a network.

   D. Any device that connects to Wi-Fi.

CORRECT ANSWERS AND RATIONALES

1. B. ASCII
2. A. A wave's peak is considered a binary 1, and a wave's trough is considered a binary 0.
3. D. An electronic envelop used to transmit information over the network.
4. B. To detect network traffic and collisions of packets.
5. A. 2.
6. A. A device connected to the network.
7. B. The transfer of packets between networks.
8. D. Network broadcast.
9. A. Emails remain on the email server.
10. C. Any device that can interact with a network.

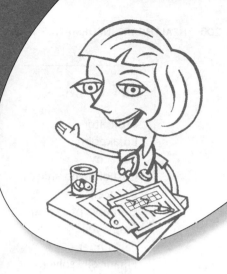

chapter **8**

Clinical Vendor Negotiations

KEY TERMS

Arbitrator	Negotiation strategy
Breakpoint	Payment schedule
Capacity	Penalty clause
Cost of ownership	Performance incentive
Disincentives	Proposal
Elements of a contract	Regulatory compliance
Employee	Request for information
Fact finder	Request for proposal
Financially solvent	Risks of procurement
General contractor	Stages of adoption
Goods	Uniform Commercial Code
Industry standards	Vendor
Liability	Zero sum game
Mediator	

Many direct and indirect tasks are required to provide patient care. Direct tasks are tasks that can be directly associated with patient outcomes such as nursing care, medications, and accommodations in the patient's room. An indirect task is a task that is in support of a direct task such as hiring the nurse, acquiring medication, and procuring and maintaining the electronic medical records application.

A task, regardless if the task is a direct or indirect task is performed by a resource. The resource can be an **employee** of the healthcare facility or a **vendor**, sometimes referred to as a contractor. For example, a healthcare facility can use employees to build and maintain an electronic medical records application or purchase an electronic medical records application from a vendor and engage the vendor to maintain the application.

There is a clear distinction between an employee and a vendor. Tasks performed by an employee are controlled by the healthcare facility. Administrators determine what tasks need to be done, when to do the tasks, and how to perform the tasks. Every detail of the task is controlled by administrators.

In contrast, the healthcare facility has practically no influence on the details of tasks beyond an agreement with a vendor. Administrators engage a vendor to produce an outcome of tasks such as to implement electronic medical records systems. Administrators specify conditions within which the vendor produces the outcome such as the time frame, cost, and access to the healthcare facility and other constraints. However, the vendor controls every aspect of all tasks that are necessary to achieve the desired outcome. The vendor hires vendor employees, engages other vendors, commonly called subcontractors, and determines work schedules and work rules.

The nurse informatics specialist will be in a position to engage vendors on behalf of the healthcare facility and manage vendors throughout the length of the agreement. The nurse informatics specialist will initiate and oversee the procurement process, select vendors, negotiate with vendors, and execute a contract with the vendor. Furthermore, the nurse informatics specialist will manage the vendor during the life of the contract.

1. Procurement

Procurement is the process of acquiring **goods** and services from one or more vendors. The goal of procurement is to make the acquisition at the best possible **cost of ownership** at the right quality, quantity, place, and time and from the right vendor.

A good is an item such as an electronic medical records application. A service is something that is done for you—an outcome—such as a vendor implementing the electronic medical records application. Think of a service as performing a task.

Cost of ownership is the total cost of acquiring and using a good or service. This includes development, implementation, and maintenance. Development is the effort to get the item ready to use. Implementation is the effort to install the item, and maintenance is the ongoing effort to continue to use the item.

For the electronic medical record system, development includes acquiring new computers, upgrading the network, redesign of workflows, and training. Implementation is overtime for installing and testing the electronic medical records application. Maintenance is ongoing support for the electronic medical records application that includes hiring specialist to oversee the application. Also included are the cost of electricity, maintenance of computers that run the application, and the maintenance agreement with the vendor. All costs are estimated before choosing a vendor.

Procurement Process

The procurement process begins when the healthcare facility identifies a need. Needs are prioritized by the administration. Those with the highest priority are assigned to a project manager to meet those needs. The term *project manager* is a functional title that describes a person who is responsible for addressing the need. That is, the person may have a title other than project manager such as nurse informatics specialist.

The initial step in the procurement process is a needs assessment. A needs assessment is the process of clearly identifying the outcome such as automating medical records. Needs must be specific. That is, what medical records need to be automated, and what is meant by automation? Answering these and similar questions in the needs assessment is challenging because each of us generally knows what is meant by automating medical records, yet our expectations are likely to be different from each other. The needs assessment must explicitly identify stakeholder expectations. Furthermore, the needs assessment must include requirements of regulatory agencies such as meaningful use (see Chapter 1).

The project manager must be able to express in writing the specific need to vendors who might be able to fulfill those needs. If the need cannot be expressed in writing, then it is not the right time to make the procurement. That is, if the project manager does not know what is needed, then how will a vendor know what is needed?

Finding a Vendor

The next step in the procurement process is finding a vendor that can meet the need. The goal is to identify a small group of qualified vendors, each of whom can submit a **proposal** to meet the need to the project manager. A qualified vendor is a vendor that can provide the need within the requirements set forth by the healthcare facility.

Here are a few common qualifications:

- **Financially solvent**: The vendor must have the financial resources to be self-supporting during the project. A vendor is typically paid upon delivery of the need (i.e., successful implementation of the electronic medical record system), although some procurement arrangements require progress payments. A progress payment is an amount paid by the healthcare facility to the vendor at designated milestones in the project. All expenses incurred by the vendor leading up to delivering the need are financed by the vendor. If the vendor lacks financial stability, then the vendor may be unable to pay its expenses and therefore will be unable to complete the project.

- Existing relationship: A vendor that successfully meets other needs of the healthcare facility should be considered for the project if the vendor has the expertise to fulfill the need. The healthcare facility and the vendor have a comfortable working relationship with each other.

- Expertise: The vendor must know how to provide the need. Some needs are highly specialized such as implementing the Epic electronic medical record system. (Epic is a major provider of electronic medical record systems.) A vendor may be knowledgeable on the implementation of a McKesson electronic medical record system (McKesson is another major provider of electronic medical record systems) but has never implemented an Epic electronic medical record system and lacks the necessary expertise. However, some needs can be met by many vendors such as printing training material.

- Experience: Do not confuse experience with expertise. Expertise is the knowledge to do something, and experience is having applied that knowledge many times. A highly desirable vendor is one who has met the exact needs required by the healthcare facility many times for other similar healthcare facilities. Similarities are based on size, specialty, patient demographics, revenue source, and other factors that distinguish healthcare facilities.

- **General contractor** vs. integrated contractor: A general contractor is a vendor that takes on the responsibility to meet the need and will likely hire other vendors called subcontractors to perform some or all tasks needed to fulfill the need. An integrated contractor is a vendor that takes on the responsibility to meet the need and will perform all tasks needed to fulfill the need. Both types of vendors can meet the healthcare facility's need.

- **Capacity:** The vendor must have the capacity to fulfill the need within the time frame specified by the healthcare facility. A vendor may be financially solvent and has the necessary expertise and experience but has too many obligations with other clients. That is, the vendor lacks the capacity to take on the healthcare facility's project.

After the vendor qualifications are identified, the next step is to locate vendors. Review current and past vendors who have done business with the healthcare facility to determine if they might be qualified for the project. Speak with counterparts in other healthcare facilities who have had similar needs to determine vendors considered for their project and the vendor selected for their project. Contact vendors who worked for the healthcare facility on similar projects. They may be able to recommend candidates. Professional associations are also good resource for suggesting vendors.

> **NURSING ALERT**
>
> Google and other web sources can be used to find a vendor, but a personal search will likely find viable candidates in the shortest time period.

Contacting Vendors

Next prepare a **request for information** document that can be sent to prospective vendors. The request for information document provides general information about the needs of the healthcare facility and requests information about the vendor and the vendor's products and services.

A representative of the vendor may follow up personally to begin discussions about the project. Discussion should focus on verifying the vendor's qualification and providing generalized information about the project. Project specifications will be sent to selected vendors in a formal document called a **request for proposal**.

Some vendors may not be interested in the project for a variety of reasons, including that the vendor does not feel qualified to meet the need. A vendor may decide that the project is too small or too big for the vendor. The vendor may also decide to pass because there is not enough profit for the vendor in the project or the vendor does not like doing business with the healthcare facility.

There are two outcomes from the request for information. First, the project manager learns from vendors more information about the realities of meeting the need. Initially, administrators and the project manager may think this is a relatively straightforward project but realize the complexity of the project after speaking with vendors. For example, the network infrastructure of the healthcare facility might need upgrading to support the electronic medical record system. The other outcome is weeding of the vendor list both by vendors who think the project is not right for them and by the project manager who determines that a vendor is not a good candidate for the project.

The Proposal

After information is received from vendors and verified for accuracy (vetted), the project manager creates a request for proposal, sometimes referred to as request for quotation. The request contains specific information about the project, including expectations, timeline, and constraints. Expectations are specific outcomes. Constraints are limitations within which those outcomes are to be achieved. It is critical to be specific in the request for proposal because this is the information that the vendor will use to propose how the vendor is going to meet the healthcare facility's needs. The request for proposal must state a deadline when proposals are due.

The vendor will submit a proposal to the project manager. The proposal is a description of how the vendor is going to meet the need based on information in the request for proposal. The proposal should contain the price to be paid to the vendor; however, some vendors may prefer to omit the price to give the vendor leverage in negotiations.

Do not review proposals until after the deadline specified in the request for proposal. The project manager should assemble a committee of appropriate stakeholders to review all proposals. The review should consider:

- Completeness: The proposal should address all specifications mentioned in the request for proposal. Be alert. Some vendors address a few but not all specifications. The reasons for submitting a partial proposal are many. Regardless of the reason, the vendor that submits an incomplete proposal is indicating noncompliance with the healthcare facility's request.

- Specificity: The proposal should address requested specification in sufficient detail so that committee members can comprehend the nature of the proposal.

- Restatements: Statements of requirements mentioned in the request for proposal should remain unchanged in the proposal. Some vendors may reword the statement, leading to vagueness in the requirements that were clear in the proposal. For example, the request for proposal may state that the vendor will provide an electronic medical record system that includes electronic medication administration record, order management, and computer practitioner order entry. The proposal might state that the vendor will provide an electronic medical record system and not mention components specified in the request for proposal. Time, price, and other elements of the proposal may not reflect those components.

- Authorization: The proposal must be submitted under the name of the company representative who has authority to submit a proposal. For example, a sales representative may not have authority to submit binding proposals.

- Feasibility: The committee must determine if the proposal is feasible. If all but one proposal extends the timeline mentioned in the request for proposal and the cost is 30% less than other proposals, then there is a question of whether it is feasible for that vendor to fulfill the terms of the proposal.

The goal of the committee is to select two or three of the most promising vendors for a more thorough review. The review entails personal interviews, sampling each vendor's product or service, visits to vendor clients, and other activities that provide detailed information to the committee about the vendor.

One vendor is then selected, and negotiations begin between the healthcare facility and the vendor (see Negotiations).

Risks of Procurement

On the surface, most or all responsibility and related risks associated with fulfilling the healthcare facility's need is shifted from the healthcare facility to the vendor. If the vendor is contracted to implement an electronic medical records system, then the vendor is responsible for the implementation. All risks associated with the implementation are borne by the vendor.

In reality, the healthcare facility also remains exposed to those risk. Although the healthcare facility may withhold payment to the vendor for nondelivery, the need of the healthcare facility remains unfulfilled. Repercussions for not fulfilling the need such as regulatory obligations must be handled by the healthcare facility. Therefore, administrators must monitor a vendor carefully during the project.

There are common areas where procurement is likely to fail. These are:

- Unclear statement of work: The request for proposal and proposal do not specify all the details of the work and therefore appear less complex than the work is.

- Overstatement of work: The request for proposal and therefore the proposal is too specific, not giving the vendor sufficient flexibility to deliver what the healthcare facility needs, not what they want.

- Communication breakdown: Specifications that are costly or impracticable in the request for proposal are pointed out by the vendor but are not changed and remain in the proposal.

- Poor diligence: The committee did not verify everything in the vendor proposal, resulting in a proposal that favors the vendor over the healthcare facility.

- No basis for price: The proposal should specify how the vendor arrived at the total price for the project, providing a foundation for the committee to understand the pricing of the project.

- One-sided proposal: Either the healthcare provider or the vendor has self-serving terms that are not negotiable.

2. Negotiation

Negotiation is the process of two or more parties reaching an agreement. The negotiation process can be as simple as two people agreeing to meet at a specific time and place or as complex as a labor contract between the healthcare facility and the bargaining unit. The nurse informatics specialist in the role of project manager will likely be required to negotiate contracts with vendors to provide various services to the healthcare facility.

Negotiations with a vendor can be as simple as agreeing on a price to print training material supplied by nurse informatics specialists or as complex as acquiring the rights to use an electronic medical records application. The complexity of negotiations is determined by the complexity of the product or service that the vendor provides and the impact that the product or service has on the healthcare facility.

For example, implementing an electronic medical records application not only requires acquisition and installation of the software application but also many other factors. These include:

- **Liability**: Liability will be incurred if the electronic medical records application malfunctions, resulting in injury or death of a patient because of inappropriate medical treatment based on the patient's electronic medical record.

- Data: Information collected by the electronic medical records application is stored in a database maintained by the vendor. The healthcare facility and the vendor must agree as to who owns the data. The patient owns the patient's medical record; however, the healthcare facility owns the format of the data.

- Accessing data: Data collected by the electronic medical records application can be accessed using the application. The healthcare facility and the vendor must decide if the healthcare facility can directly access the data from the database, bypassing the application. This may be important for the healthcare facility if the healthcare facility was to generate reports that are not available in the application.

- Transferring data: The healthcare facility should determine how data can be transferred to a different electronic medical records application if the healthcare facility decides to terminate the agreement with the vendor.

- **Regulatory compliance**: Standards required by regulatory authorities are typically incorporated into the electronic medical records application. The healthcare facility and the vendor must agree that the vendor will ensure that the application is always regulatory compliant.

- Price: Both parties must agree on what is and what is not covered in the price of the electronic medical records application. Likewise, there should be agreement on a pricing structure for items not covered under the quoted price. For example, minor upgrades are covered, but major upgrades are not. Guidelines for prices should be included when the agreement is renewed such as no more than a 10% increase in price.

- Termination: All agreements end. The goal is to agree on an amiable termination arrangement during negotiations. This includes not renewing the agreement; breach of the agreement; and if the vendor is sold, merged, or goes out of business.

> **NURSING ALERT**
>
> The healthcare facility provides the nurse informatics specialist support during vendor negotiations that include an attorney.

Preparing for Negotiations

Complex negotiations require a strategy similar to a chess game in which there are a gambit (opening move), countermoves, testing the opponent in midgame strategy, and then developing the end game-winning move. Chess is a **zero sum game**. That is, there is a winner and a loser. No one wins in a tie.

Negotiation is not a zero sum game—and there are no ties. Instead, each party wins something and loses something. The goal for both sides is to win elements that are important. For example, the price must reflect a reasonable profit for the vendor. Both sides negotiate to define reasonable. There is a price point when the vendor will walk away from the negotiation because there is no sufficient profit to be made on the project. There is a price point when the healthcare facility is unwilling or unable to pay and will walk away from negotiations. If both sides cannot define a reasonable price, then there is no purchase.

Preparation is the first step in the negotiation process. Preparation will identify:

- Required factors: Required factors are factors that are not negotiable. If those factors are not in the final agreement, then there is no agreement, and the healthcare facility will walk away from negotiations. For example, the electronic medical records application must be compliant and remain compliant with regulatory authorities.

- Negotiable factors: Negotiable factors are factors that are nice to have but will not stop the healthcare facility from agreeing with the vendor. For example, the electronic medical records application is fully integrated with the electronic medical records application, order management application, and computer practitioner order entry application. However, the healthcare facility will accept a partially integrated system.

- Not required factors: Not required factors are factors that are unimportant to the healthcare facility. For example, the healthcare facility is not a member of the vendor's customer advisory committee.

Preparation will also assess the same factors for the vendor—that is, required factors, negotiable factors, and not required factors for the vendor. The assessment is not perfect but will provide a rationale for developing a **negotiation strategy**. Know the worth of the project to the vendor and to the healthcare facility. Does the vendor need the healthcare facility more than the healthcare facility needs the vendor? The answer to this question determines which side is negotiating from strength.

After factors are identified for both sides of the negotiation, the healthcare facility focuses on developing a negotiation strategy—a strategy for each stage of negotiations. The healthcare facility's negotiating team plots moves. The vendor's proposal is the opening gambit for the vendor. The healthcare facility's negotiating team determines a counterproposal and projects the vendor's possible reactions to the counterproposal.

The outcome of the planning process is a well-thought-out plan for negotiation.

NURSING ALERT

No negotiation strategy is perfect. Unanticipated actions by the vendor can set any well-designed plan into turmoil. Therefore, the negotiating team must remain flexible throughout the negotiation process.

Negotiation Strategy

Decide your **breakpoint**. The breakpoint is the least terms that are acceptable to the healthcare facility such as required factors. Next, open with an extreme position that is far above the breakpoint. These are required factors and are presented as non- negotiable. The worst that can happen is that the vendor returns with a counteroffer.

The difference between the healthcare facility's initial offer and the vendor's counteroffer is the bargaining range. A settlement will be reached somewhere within this range. Therefore, it is important to make the initial offer as extreme as possible to give the healthcare facility sufficient room for negotiation.

Negotiations should incrementally narrow the bargaining range. Each increment should be perceived as a major concession regardless of the actual importance of the factors negotiated.

Identify incentives and **disincentives**. An incentive is something of value to the vendor that can be offered if the vendor performs certain actions. For example, the vendor will receive a 10% increase over the negotiated price if the project is delivered fully operational 6 months ahead of the schedule. Of course, all specifications must be met.

A disincentive is a penalty for the vendor for not adhering to specific terms of the contract. For example, the healthcare facility will penalize the vendor 1% of the price for each month over the scheduled deadline.

NURSING ALERT

A disincentive typically specifies conditions related to the lack of action such as the penalty is voided if the healthcare facility materially alters the original specifications.

Value

Value is the perception of worth. The perception of value is used in negotiation to create a relatively low-cost incentive to reach terms of a contract. Let's say that a vendor that supplies computing equipment offers the healthcare facility printers at a reasonable cost if the healthcare facility contracts with the vendor to supply computers for the entire facility at market value. That is, other vendors can provide the same computers at relatively the same price.

The vendor perceives that printers are having a relatively low value because the vendor has many printers in inventory. Yet the healthcare facility views printers as a high value because the printers are being acquired at what is perceived as below market value.

The negotiating teams should evaluate perceptions of value when deciding to negotiate incentives.

Do the Math

A good negotiator will estimate how much it will cost to provide the product or service that is being negotiated. Let's say that the vendor is going to charge $8000 for 4 days of one onsite support person during the first 4 days that the electronic medical record system goes live. Is this a good deal?

One way to assess the value of this support is to estimate the expenses that the vendor incurs when sending the representative to the healthcare facility's location. These expenses include the cost of air travel; cabs to and from the airport; the hotel stay; a reasonable amount for meals; transportation to and from the healthcare facility's site; and the salary and benefits paid to the employee.

Calculating the cost gives a rough estimate of whether the $8000 is reasonable. This also serves as a basis for negotiation. The vendor may be willing to lower the price because it perceives the value as being relatively low. That is, the employee's compensation is being paid whether or not the employee is onsite or in the office. Therefore, the vendor may be willing to waive part of the $8000 that is part of the employee's compensation. However, any reduction would not be put forth unless the healthcare facility estimates the cost.

> ### NURSING ALERT
>
> Superstores that offer extremely low prices calculate every cost associated with products purchased from vendors. The superstore knows how much it costs to make the product. They leverage this knowledge to negotiate low prices from vendors that supply the product. In essence, the superstore knows terms that make the deal marginally good for the vendor.

Payment

The **payment schedule** is another bargaining point. The vendor is expected to finance the project depending on the nature of the product. The healthcare facility then makes one payment to the vendor after the project is delivered and accepted.

In some projects, the vendor requires an initial payment either at contract signing or when the project begins. This is referred to as a good faith payment. The vendor may request progress payments throughout the project.

A progress payment is a portion of the total payment that the healthcare facility makes to the vendor at specific milestones during the project. The remaining payment is made when the healthcare facility accepts the delivered project. Progress payments help the vendor's cash flow during the project. Cash flow is the amount of funds paid and received. A progress payment replenishes funds that were expensed for a segment of the project.

Progress payments must be associated with delivered value. Let's say the vendor is contracted to upgrade computers, servers, and the local area network and implement an electronic medical records system for the healthcare facility.

These are segments of the project. A progress payment can be made after computers are upgraded because the vendor delivered a value to the healthcare facility. The healthcare facility has state-of-the-art computers even if nothing more is done on the project. That is, the vendor can walk away from the project, and the healthcare facility can contract with another vendor to complete the other segments of the project.

Progress payments must not be made if the vendor does not deliver value. Let's say that the vendor installed tools necessary for the nurse informatics specialist to tailor the vendor's electronic medical records system. Although this is a project deliverable, this is of no value to the healthcare facility. That is, the tools can only be used for the vendor's electronic medical record application. The tools are of no value to the healthcare facility if the vendor walks away from the project.

> ### NURSING ALERT
>
> Be sure that the vendor is economically sound before engaging the vendor. A vendor should be able to finance the entire project without progress payments.

General Contractor

A project may require a number of specialist vendors. In the example of an electronic medical record system, there is the vendor supplying the application, and there are vendors who upgrade computers, upgrade the network, upgrade servers, and train the staff to use the application. The nurse informatics specialist must decide to use a general contractor or deal directly with specialty vendors.

A general contractor is a vendor that takes on responsibility for the entire project and engages specialty contractors to complete their portions of the contract. Specialty contractors engaged by a general contractor are referred to as subcontractors. The primary benefit of using a general contractor is that the healthcare facility interacts with only one vendor. There is no need to search for specialty vendors.

There are two major disadvantages of engaging a general contractor. First, the healthcare facility has no control over subcontractors. Although the healthcare facility typically sets rules for subcontractors, the general contractor controls subcontractors. The other factor is price. The general contractor's price includes a charge for overseeing subcontractors plus a charge for each subcontractor. Typically, the price is an aggregate price for the entire project, not pricing broken down into segments (i.e., subcontractor).

The healthcare facility must weigh the options of being its own general contractor engaging each specialty vendor or engaging a general contractor. Taking on the role of the general contractor enables the healthcare facility to negotiate prices for each specialty vendor and control those vendors. However, this does not guarantee a price that is better than that given by the general contractor. The general contractor may be in a better negotiating position than the healthcare facility. For example, the general contractor has leverage that the subcontractor may work on other projects for the general contractor. The healthcare facility has one project. Furthermore, the nurse informatics specialist or another staff member must perform the duties of the general contractor.

Face-to-Face Negotiation

Face-to-face negotiations occur only when the nurse informatics specialist is prepared for negotiations. Regardless of pressures placed by the healthcare facility or the vendor, never enter negotiations unprepared. The goal of negotiations is to achieve a contract (see Contracts) that is set to terms of product or service that the vendor will provide to the healthcare facility. In theory, the vendor wants to do as little as possible to achieve the outcome while receiving the maximum amount of money for the outcome. The healthcare facility wants to achieve the best outcome while spending little money. Negotiations bring both parties to realistic terms.

Face-to-face negotiation is more about perceptions, personalities, and salesmanship than the facts of the project. Every facet of negotiations influences negotiations. An objective is to control each facet such as the site of negotiations. The negotiations site is the stage that influences perceptions. For example, the healthcare facility is perceived to be negotiating from a power of strength if negotiations are held on the healthcare facility's site, especially if discussion takes place in the chief operating officer's office. This is why negotiations for important contracts occur at a neutral place such in a hotel conference room so neither party has an advantage over the other party.

The nurse informatics specialist's behavior is critical to developing a perception of strength that you have negotiated successfully many times—even if this is your first negotiations. Speak louder than usual and greet others with a strong handshake. Lead the negotiations process. For example, say, "Thanks for coming today. Let's begin by reviewing our needs." This opening gives the impression that you are in control and the other party is following your lead.

Your body language communicates your feelings before you say a word; therefore, always maintain professional, strong body language. Sit up straight.

Maintain eye contact at all times. Display neutral or friendly facial expressions even if you are worried.

Speak with clear terms. Avoid vague terms. You need a computer practitioner's order entry system that is fully integrated with the current electronic medical records system. Never use "about," "approximately," or "it would nice to have" because this gives rise to each party defining the terms in their favor.

> ### NURSING ALERT
>
> Do not read too much into the other party's body language. A good negotiator will telegraph misleading messages using facial expressions.

Negotiating Terms

Never be the first to talk price. Price is the value placed on the product or service. Each party has its own valuation of the product or service. The first party to talk about price sets the approximate value of the product or service.

Let's say that the nurse informatics specialist is willing to pay $200,000 for the electronic medical records system. The vendor is willing to provide the system for $100,000. If the nurse informatics specialist is the first to talk price and mentions $200,000, then the vendor is likely to ask for slightly more than $200,000. The value of the product or service before either party spoke about price is unknown. The value could be $10, $10,000, $100,000, or $1 million. The first to speak about price sets the magnitude of the value.

At some point, one party breaks down and mentions price. In the theory of negotiations, the vendor's first price is higher than the eventually agreed upon price, and the healthcare facility's price is lower than the settled price.

In reality, the vendor may use a different negotiation strategy that settles for an unrealistically low price. The price put forward by a vendor is based on written specifications provided by the healthcare facility. The price reflects delivery of the specifications. However, the vendor may realize that the specifications are incomplete. That is, additional products or services are necessary to achieve the healthcare facility's outcome. The vendor proposes an attractive price, signs the contract, and begins the project. At some point during the project, the vendor and the healthcare facility realizes additional work is necessary. The vendor is in a position of strength to dictate the price for the additional work because the work is necessary, and another vendor is unlikely to bid on that work because the project is underway.

> **NURSING ALERT**
>
> It is critical that both parties explicitly state what is and what is not included in the price. Likewise, it is critical that the healthcare facility takes time to develop a complete set of specification for the project before asking for proposals.

Hold back items you want until the close of negotiations. At the end of negotiations, both parties are usually in a positive mindset, looking beyond negotiations toward starting the project. Introducing one or two items that you want included in the contract places the other party in a pressured position, and they may capitulate to those items simply to complete the negotiations.

> **NURSING ALERT**
>
> Avoid hostility leading up to and during negotiations. A party may refuse favorable terms because the party holds a grudge with the other party to the negotiations.

Terminate Negotiation

Negotiations end either with an agreement of understanding or no agreement. An agreement of understanding is a written document that contains key items that are in agreement. The agreement of understanding serves as the foundation for attorneys to draw up formal contracts. The agreement of understanding is signed before parties leave the last negotiation session. It is common that this agreement is hand written.

If no agreement can be reached after several negotiation sessions, then negotiation is terminated, and the healthcare facility seeks another vendor. The point at which negotiations terminate without an agreement of understanding is called a breakpoint. Each party determines its own breakpoint. A breakpoint is when the party walks away from negotiations because the other party is unreasonable and not negotiating in good faith.

Negotiating in good faith means that a party is sincerely interested in reaching an agreement. There are times when a party has an ulterior motive for entering into negotiations. For example, an executive in the healthcare facility may not be in favor of implementing the electronic medical records system but enters negotiations with a vendor for political purposes, making it appear that the executive is interested. In reality, the executive is not negotiating in good faith and is doing everything to encourage the vendor to terminate negotiations without an agreement.

NURSING ALERT

Large consulting firms that offer a variety of managerial and management information systems (MIS) services may provide the initial service at a very reasonable price. Employees of the consulting firm will prospect for additional work while providing the contracted service. That is, they will find other workflows not working well and offer to fix the workflow for an additional price.

---

3. Conflict Resolution

Negotiations will likely bring disagreements between the healthcare facility and the vendor. Disagreements can also occur during the project even though terms are defined in a contract. An effort should be made to resolve conflicts amicably through the conflict resolution process. The conflict resolution process helps parties focus on the factor in dispute and then try to rationalize viable options that will bring the parties to an agreement.

Disputes tend to be disproportionate to factors in agreement, resulting in distortion of the situation. Let's say the vendor successfully delivered 99% of deliverables and 1% was unacceptable, although the vendor believes it complied with specifications written in the contract. The healthcare facility and the vendor disagree that 1% of the deliverables is acceptable. Discussions focus on the unacceptable deliverable rather than reviewing the whole project. Focusing on the negative intensifies the importance of the item in dispute. The primary goal of conflict resolution is to help parties develop a balanced view of the project.

Fact Finder, Mediator, and Arbitrator

Parties to a dispute should ask a third party to intervene and help resolve the conflict. Three types of third parties can intervene in a dispute. These are:

- **Fact finder**: A fact finder is an unbiased third party whose sole purpose is to review relevant information, including contracts, performance records, **industry standards**, and other elements that influence the dispute. The fact finder assembles facts into a logical flow and presents a list of facts to both parties. The parties use the list of facts as a starting point to renegotiate the conflict.

- **Mediator**: A mediator is an unbiased third party who is trained to mediate disputes. The goal of a mediator is to help both parties to resolve the conflict. The mediator begins with fact finding and then interviews each party separately and confidentially to understand the situation and the party's concern. The mediator tries to find a middle ground and options that are acceptable to both parties. The mediator does not resolve the dispute; rather, both parties resolve the dispute with the help of the mediator.

- **Arbitrator**: An arbitrator is also an unbiased third party; however, an arbitrator—not the disputing parties—resolves the dispute in a process called arbitration. That is, an arbitrator is judge and jury. Each party submits facts and their positions to the arbitrator in person, in writing, or both. The arbitrator makes a judgment, and the dispute is resolved. There are two types of arbitration. These are nonbinding and binding. Nonbinding arbitration occurs when the decision of the arbitrator can be rejected by either or both parties. Binding arbitration occurs when the decision of the arbitrator legally binds both parties. Both parties must accept the resolution.

Suing

Disputes related to contracts are usually not brought to court to resolve the dispute. Although each party to a contract dispute has the right to sue, suing is not practical. In addition to legal costs, it can be years before the parties appear before a judge. The impact to the project is devastating by that time. Both parties win—and both lose.

Binding arbitration is the preferred route over suing in court because the parties can be heard before an arbitrator within weeks rather than years. The arbitrator is likely to be a retired judge or lawyer who applies many of the same practices found in court. The issue can be expedited within a reasonable time period and limited impact on the project.

A contract (see Contracts) usually has a clause that states that all contract disputes will be resolved in binding arbitration. Parties who sign a contract that contains the binding arbitration clause are obligated by law to agree to the judgment of the arbitrator. Furthermore, parties agree to waive their right to bring the dispute to court.

The List

A disagreement is typically small, although a small disagreement can stop the parties from agreeing on an overall contract. The mediator's role is to illustrate to both parties exactly what is in disagreement. In this way, the parties may see a balanced view of issues affecting the project. More times than not, both parties are in agreement. It is just that the disagreement overshadows items that are in agreement.

The mediator lists all items in agreement on a legal pad or on a white board. The objective is to make this list visibly long. The list is assembled from fact finding conducted by the mediator before bringing both sides together to review the mediator's findings. The mediator presents a fact and asks each party if they are in agreement. The mediator knows the answer because the mediator has met individually with the parties exploring the same information. Only facts that the mediator knows the parties agree on are asked and listed.

Besides the list of agreed upon items, the mediator lists items in disagreement. Again, the mediator knows the items but still asks each party for their opinions and lists the item in the second column of disagreed items. By nature and sometimes by the mediator's design, the list of disagreed items is noticeably smaller than the list of agreed items. This illustrates to the parties that they agree many more times than disagree.

Next, the mediator examines each item in disagreement and decomposes the item into subcomponents. Subcomponents are entered into two new lists—subcomponents in agreement and subcomponents in disagreement. The list of subcomponents in agreement typically is longer than those in disagreement. The process continues until there are many sets of lists, each dissecting items in disagreement, until the mediator ends with a few items that cannot be dissected further. This is the focus of the mediation.

The mediator draws a diagram of lists that pictures the magnitude of the disagreement to a very few items. In doing so, the mindset of parties in the mediation conference changes from adversaries to reasonableness. The mediator then asks each party to focus on options to resolve the remaining disagreement.

NURSING ALERT

Disagreement related to a situation with the project can likely be resolved because both parties are interested in completing the project. However, a disagreement in a deeply rooted value called a disagreement in principle is difficult to resolve because the disagreement has little or nothing to do with completing the project.

Stages of Adoption

Disputes sometimes center on the adoption process. When we ask someone to change and adopt something new, the person works through the stages of the adoption process. Each stage must be successfully completed before moving to the next stage leading to the acceptance of the change.

Let's say the vendor wants to change the other nurse informatics specialist's opinion on how the electronic medical records system should be implemented.

A dispute is likely to arise if the vendor does not give the nurse informatics specialist time to work through the **stages of adoption**. That is, the vendor wants the nurse informatics specialist to make a decision quickly. The nurse informatics specialist is likely to resist, leading to a dispute.

There are five stages of adoption. These are:

- Awareness: In the awareness stage, the nurse informatics specialist becomes aware of a possible solution to a problem involving implementation of the electronic medical records system. The solution is proposed by the vendor.

- Exploration: In the exploration stage, the nurse informatics specialist takes a superficial look at the solution to determine if this is a possible solution.

- Examination: In the examination stage, the nurse informatics specialist takes a detailed look at the possible solutions to uncover reasons why the solution will fail.

- Test: In the test stage, the nurse informatics specialist tries the solution under various scenarios to assess whether or not the solution is viable.

- Adoption: In the adoption stage, the nurse informatics specialist consults with the vendor that the solution will solve the problem with the implementation of the electronic medical records system.

To avoid disputes, the vendor must give the nurse informatics specialist time to work through each stage of adoption. The vendor can assist by providing the nurse informatics specialist resources, information, and other facts that help assess each stage.

4. Contract

A contract is an agreement between two or more persons to do something or to refrain from doing something in exchange for something of value called consideration. A person is a legal entity such as an individual, partnership, or corporation.

A legal entity is an organization, such as a vendor, that has the right to act as a person. Individuals form a legal entity to conduct business and limit liability. Liability is the risk associated with conducting business. For example, the vendor is liable for performing the terms of the contract. Failure to do so provides a reason to the healthcare facility to take legal action against the vendor, placing the vendor's assets (property and money) at risk.

An individual is a legal entity who can conduct business. The individual pays all expenses associated with the business and receives all revenues generated by the business. The individual is also personally liable to fulfill obligations stated in a contract with a customer. The individual manages the business.

A partnership is another legal entity. A partnership is formed by two or more individuals who work toward a common goal such as providing a product or service to earn a profit. Each partner provides value to the partnership in the form of assets (money or property). Partners then share the revenues and profits realized by the partnership.

There are two types of partnerships. These are a general partnership and a limited liability partnership (LLP). In a general partnership, each partner is responsible for the liability of the partnership. That is, a general partner's personal assets can be used by creditors to pay the liabilities of the partnership. An LLP legally limits a partner's liability to the partner's investment in the partnership. The limited liability partner's personal assets cannot be used by creditors to pay the liability of the partnership. Each partner participates in managing the business based on the partnership agreement. The partnership agreement specifies terms of the partnership. That is, one partner may manage the business (managing partner), and other partners are advisors. Alternatively, all partners manage the business.

A corporation is also a legal entity authorized by the government to act as person formed by individuals called stockholders. Stockholders provide the corporation with assets—usually money—in exchange for shares of stock. Each share has the right to receive a portion of profits generated by the corporation. Profits are distributed per share. Stockholders elect a board of directors that hires individuals to manage the business. A stockholder does not manage the business.

Elements of a Contract

There are two types of contracts. These are:

- Oral contract: An oral contract is a verbal agreement between two parties that contains all the **elements of a contract**. Although terms of the agreement are not written, the contract is enforceable under the law. However, the Statue of Fraud specifies that some contracts such as for real estate must be written.

- Written contract: A written contract is a document that contains terms of an agreement between two parties. Contracts between the healthcare facility and vendors are typically written contracts.

Every contract must have four elements. An agreement that does not have these four elements is not a contract. These are:

- Offer: An offer is the promise to act or refrain from acting sometimes in the future.

- Consideration: Consideration is something of value promised to the party who makes the offer. The value can be money, a product, or a service.

- Acceptance: Acceptance is the action that clearly agrees to the offer. Acceptance can be conveyed in words, deeds, or performance in accordance with terms of the offer. Actions contrary to the offer can be construed as rejecting the offer or making a counteroffer. Acceptance must occur within a reasonable time.

- Mutuality: Mutuality means that both parties to the contract understood the terms of the contract when the contract was signed.

During negotiations, each party can make an offer. When an offer is made, the other party can accept or make a counteroffer. When a counteroffer is made, the offer is no longer valid. That is, the party who rejects the offer cannot accept the offer when a counteroffer is made. Let's say that the vendor offers to implement an electronic medical records system to perform a specified functionality for $100,000. The healthcare facility proposes a counteroffer for additional functionality for $90,000, which is rejected by the vendor. At this point, no offer is on the table. The healthcare facility cannot say, "Okay, I'll take it for $100,000" and expect the vendor to be obligated to return to the original offer.

> **NURSING ALERT**
>
> A gift is to transfer something of value without receiving something (consideration) in return for the transfer.

Breach of Contract

A breach of contract occurs when one party to the contract fails to perform some or all terms of the contract without legal cause. There are two types of breach of contract. These are:

- Material breach: A material breach occurs when the other party receives something substantially different than that specified in the contract. A material breach occurs if the electronic medical records system does not perform as specified in the contract.

- Minor breach: A minor breach occurs when the other party receives substantial things specified in the contract. Let's say that the contract calls for the vendor to implement the electronic medical records system by a specific date and the system was implemented 2 weeks late. The healthcare facility received the electronic medical records system substantially late.

A breach of contract is not enforceable if there is a legal cause to breach the contract, which is commonly referred to as a defense to the breach of contract. Common legal causes are:

- Illegal: Actions specified in the contract are contrary to law such as committing a crime.

- An element missing: The contract lacked one or more of the four elements of a contract.

- Mutual mistake: The contract contains terms that both parties misunderstood.

- Unilateral mistake: One party to the contract agreed to what is an obvious mistake and the other party knew or should have known of the mistake.

- Fraud: One party obtained the agreement fraudulently.

- Performance is impossible: A party is unable to perform a requirement of the contract. Let's say that the vendor is to implement an electronic medical records system by a specific date, but the healthcare facility does not have the necessary computing devices in place; and therefore, the vendor is in breach of contract.

- Lack of capacity: A party to the contract is not of legal age or is mentally incompetent to enter into a contract.

NURSING ALERT

Failure to perform according to industry standards is a violation of a contract even though the standard is not defined in the contract.

Contract Interpretation

A contract is composed of words and phrases, either spoken or written. Both parties must have a good understanding of the meaning of those words and phrases. Any misunderstanding that is not resolved before the contract is signed can lead to a material or minor breach of the contract—and discourse between the healthcare facility and the vendor.

Properly written contracts by an attorney define key words and phrases at the beginning of the contract to reduce any misunderstanding. However, no matter how carefully written a contract, there always seems room for misinterpretation. Each party might be able to honestly arrive at a different interpretation for the same word or phrase.

Contract disputes are commonly resolved by an arbitrator or the courts by the arbitrator or judge determining the meaning of the word or phrase. The decision is based on the entire contract and the ordinary meaning of the word or phrase. That is, the arbitrator or judge initially looks at the parties' intentions by comparing elements of the contract and the performance of each party. Focus then turns on the customary usage of the term within the community (i.e., specific business or location).

The Uniform Commercial Code

The **Uniform Commercial Code** (UCC) is a recommendation of laws that states should adopt to promote uniformity of commercial laws throughout the United States. The UCC was developed by the American Law Institute and the National Conference of Commissioners on Uniform State Laws.

The goal is to create a set of rules for commercial transactions. Rules for commerce are set in law by each state. Issues can arise over commercial transactions that cross state lines. Conflicts can be avoided if each state adopts the UCC as state law.

The UCC defines rules for the sales of goods, leases, negotiable instruments, banking, letters of credit, auctions, liquidations, title documents, and securities. Furthermore, the UCC contains recommendations for formation of a contract.

Warranty

Products or services provided by a vendor are covered under a warranty. A warranty means that the vendor provides assurance that the healthcare facility will receive the desired outcome. For example, the electronic medical records system will maintain patients' medical records according to the specification in the contract. If expectations are not met, then the vendor will remedy the situation.

There is an implied warranty granted by the vendor even if a warranty is not mentioned in the contract. An implied warranty means that the vendor by the nature of the agreement assures that the product or service will meet the promised outcome. For example, the electronic medical records system is expected to maintain patients' medical records by the nature that this is the purpose of the application.

A limited warranty is a warranty defined in the contract. For example, the vendor may specify that a computing device has a 30-day warranty. After 30 days, the healthcare facility is responsible for parts and labor if the computing device fails. All terms of the warranty are written in the contract.

A warranty covers normal wear and tear on the product. If the healthcare facility abuses the product by not following the manufacturer's recommended usage, then the warranty is voided. Likewise, the warranty will not cover acts of God or malicious destruction. An act of God is an event that occurs outside of anyone's control such as a natural disaster.

An extended warranty may be available from the vendor or from an insurer to cover events that are excluded from the conventional warranty. The healthcare facility must carefully weigh likely occurrence with the expense of the extended warranty.

Remedies

A breach of contract can be remedied by the party that breached the contract by providing compensation to the other party. This is commonly referred to as damages. There are two types of damages. These are:

- Compensatory damages: Compensatory damages return the other party to whole. That is, the party that breached the contract gives the other party compensation to make up for the party's actual loss. Let's say that the electronic medical records system's malfunction caused the healthcare facility to use a paper backup system. The cost of implementing the paper backup system is considered compensatory damages.

- Punitive damages: Punitive damages punish the party that breached the contract. Punitive damages are also known as exemplary damages. For example, a vendor that abandons the implementation of the electronic medical records system halfway through the project may be punished by the arbitrator or judge for this intentional act.

NURSING ALERT

Both compensatory and punitive damages can be awarded, but settlements are usually reached by both parties for less than the awarded amount because of legal expenses related to appealing the decision.

Remedies are commonly written in the contract to avoid litigation. Both parties anticipate common reasons for breach of contract and agree to remedies that will automatically be implemented if a breach occurs. For example, the vendor agrees to compensate the healthcare facility for patient medical records that are lost because of a malfunction of the electronic medical records system.

A certain amount in dollars may be specified, or a formula for calculating that amount may be included in the agreement. A remedy might be written in the contract as a certain dollar amount or a formula for calculating the dollar amount.

Modifying a Contract

A contract can be modified with mutual consent at any time after the contract is signed. Minor modifications are written as an addendum to the existing contract and placed at the end of the contract. Major modifications typically require the reopening of negotiations.

Modifications must take into considerations that one or both parties have begun work on the project based on the terms in the existing contract. Modifications should not attempt to alter completed or partially completed work unless both parties consider such change reasonable.

Memorandum of Understanding

A memorandum of understanding is a written agreement that clarifies an understanding between two parties. A memorandum of understanding may or may not be a contract depending on the structure of the memorandum. If the memorandum has all the elements of a contract (see Elements of a Contract), then the memorandum is a contract and is enforceable.

A memorandum missing at least one element of a contract is not a contract and therefore is not enforceable. However, the memorandum may be used to show the intention of both parties to an arbitrator or judge.

Contract Termination

A contract terminates when the conditions of the contract are met by both parties or when both parties mutually agree to terminate the contract prior to meeting the contracted conditions. The contract can be terminated by mutual consent at any time.

A contract may contain a termination clause. A termination clause is a portion of the contract that specifies when the contract can be terminated and terms of how parties will be compensated, if necessary.

5. Working the Contract

A contract is a working document during the life of the project and contains all of the items agreed upon between the vendor and the healthcare facility. Both parties must manage the project within the terms of the contract.

Neither party has the right to deviate from the intent and the letter of the contract. The intent of the contract is the overall purpose of the contract as defined by words and phrases within the contract. For example, the intent is that the vendor and the healthcare facility will implement the electronic medical records system for the healthcare facility. The letter of the contract refers to the words and phrases used in the contract. For example, the contract might state that the vendor may substitute materials. The term may mean that the vendor—not the healthcare facility—has the option. Both the intent and letter of the contract must be followed during the project. Failure to do so results in a breach of contract (see Breach of Contract) that may lead to termination of the contract and damages.

Each party fulfills its obligations specified in the contract according to the party's interpretation of the contract. Ideally, both parties have the same interpretation. In reality, both parties agree to a reasonable interpretation. That is, the interpretation may differ, but generally the interpretation is the same. For example, the contract may state that the vendor will deliver an item on a specific date. The vendor interprets this as an approximate date defined as the week of the specified date. The healthcare facility interprets this as the specific date; however, the vendor's interpretation is acceptable because the item was delivered within a reasonable time period.

Reasonableness

Reasonableness plays an important factor in a working relationship between parties. Although a contract is legally binding, a contract is a goal with conditions to reach the goal. In reality, sometimes those conditions are not practical, which is not known until the project is underway. Therefore, both parties must use reasonableness when confronted by conditions that differ from conditions specified in the contract.

Let's say that the vendor is late in delivering an item based on conditions in the contract. Technically, the vendor breached the contract. The healthcare facility has a choice to terminate the contract or continue with the contract. Termination may not be the best choice because it would delay achieving the goal of the contract. Although the delay violated terms of the contract and frustrates administrators of the healthcare facility, reasonableness dictates that the contract continues and the delay is accepted.

Minor breaches of the contract maybe overlooked as long as the project is on track and will eventually produce the desired outcome. Major breaches of the contract need to be analyzed carefully before the course of action is decided.

Industry Standard

Although the terms of a contract govern the performance of each party to the contract, a vendor is obligated to perform according to industry standards. Industry standard is either a formal rule set forth by a regulatory authority or by a professional organization or a practice widely accepted in the business community.

Let's say the healthcare facility's maintenance department orders wood to build desks for a nursing station. The order is placed with the lumber company for "150 pieces of two by four." This refers to 2 feet by 4 feet. The delivered pieces are 1 ¾ feet by 3 ½ feet. The measurement delivered is different than the measurement ordered, yet the delivered wood meets industry standards; therefore, the vendor complied with the terms of the contract.

Industry standard is either implied or explicit in a contract. In the lumber example, industry standard is implied. Both parties are expected to know the industry standard and understand that meeting the standard is acceptable performance of the contract. Industry standard is explicitly mentioned in a contract to define expectations for the deliverable. For example, the contract stipulates that the electronic medical records system meets The Joint Commission standards. The Joint Commission standards become an enforceable part of the contract terms.

NURSING ALERT

Always inquire about industry standards that might apply to the contract during negotiations with the vendor. The vendor may assume there is a mutual understanding that industry standards will apply without explicitly mentioning those standards.

Penalty Clause and Performance Incentives

Financial disincentives and incentives can be included in a contract to encourage desirable performance by the vendor. A financial disincentive commonly referred to as a **penalty clause** reduces compensation to the vendor for failure to comply with terms of the contract. For example, the vendor's compensation will be reduced by 1% per month each month beyond the deadline. The penalty clause is considered an agreed upon remedy for a breach of contract related to missed deadline.

A **performance incentive**, commonly referred to as a performance incentive clause, is additional compensation provided to the vendor for desirable performance as defined by the healthcare facility. For example, the vendor's compensation will increase by 1% per month each month ahead of schedule. The value of the performance incentive clause should correspond to a financial benefit to the healthcare facility such as reduced staff overtime cost. If there is no financial benefit, then there should not be a performance incentive. That is, if the healthcare facility is not saving money or increasing revenue by having the electronic medical records system implemented earlier than the deadline, then there is no rationale for increasing compensation to the vendor for delivering before the deadline.

The Contract Manager

There should be one person designated as the contract manager, sometimes referred to as the clerk of the works. The contract manager is responsible for ensuring that terms of the contract are being met during the life of the project.

The contract manager monitors deliverables, facilitates the vendor working on site, coordinates resolution of conflicts between the vendor and the healthcare facility, and verifies that deliverables meet contract requirements. The contract manager is authorized by the healthcare facility to accept deliverables on behalf of the healthcare facility. When the contract manager signs an acceptance memorandum, the vendor's obligation to perform is completed.

Service-Level Agreement

A service-level agreement (SLA) defines the minimum service that a vendor will provide to the healthcare facility. Minimum service is measured in various ways depending on the nature of the service. The vendor is expected to meet the minimum service levels; otherwise, the healthcare facility may consider the contract breached, and remedies might be implemented.

If the service is for equipment, the minimum service is defined as mean time between failures (MTBF), mean time to repair, or mean time to recovery (MTTR). MTBF is the period when the equipment is expected to be operational. Equipment manufacturers test equipment to determine when the equipment is likely to fail. Manufacturers recommend preventive maintenance to occur before the project failure. Mean time to repair is the time that transpires between when the vendor is notified of the failure to the time when the equipment is operational again. MTTR is similar to mean time to repair except the operational downtime is likely caused by equipment failure, software failure, or a combination of factors, not simply equipment failure.

CASE STUDY

CASE 1

More than 1 year ago, the healthcare facility entered into an agreement with a vendor to implement an electronic medical records system. The vendor is a reputable firm that has implemented similar systems in other healthcare facilities. The contract calls for the implementation to occur 3 months ago. However, this has yet to occur. The vendor has been working continually on implementation, but delays have prevented the vendor from completing the implementations. As the nurse informatics specialist and project manager, the chief nursing officer asks you the following questions. What are your best responses?

QUESTION 1. Should the healthcare facility threaten to sue the vendor?

ANSWER: No. The goal of both the vendor and healthcare facility is to implement the electronic medical records system as quickly as possible. Taking legal action against the vendor will terminate the relationship with the vendor. No work will continue on the project. Furthermore, another vendor probably would not want to take over the project because the project is three-quarters complete. Any vendor that takes on the project will want to start from the beginning.

QUESTION 2. Did the vendor breach the contract?

ANSWER: A breach of contract occurrs when the vendor fails to materially implement the electronic medical records system by the deadline specified in the contract. However, if the healthcare facility's actions or inactions prevented the vendor from meeting the deadline, then the vendor has a legal defense against a breach of contract claim because the healthcare facility made it impossible for the vendor to meet the deadline.

QUESTION 3. Should we take the vendor to arbitration?

ANSWER: No. Assuming there is an arbitration clause in the contract, the arbitrator resolves conflicts between parties. There is no dispute that the vendor missed the deadline to implement the electronic medical records system. Therefore, there is no dispute to be arbitrated. However, a dispute may arise if the contract had a penalty clause that was enforced by the healthcare facility and the vendor claims that the healthcare facility prevented the vendor from meeting the deadline.

QUESTION 4. What is the best approach to take to get the vendor to implement the electronic medical records system at this point in the project?

ANSWER: Both parties need to examine the project to identify factors that are causing the delay. A joint effort must be made to overcome the barriers that prevent successful implementation of the system. The combined effort will enable the vendor to achieve the desired outcome, which is the ultimate goal of both the vendor and the healthcare facility.

FINAL CHECK-UP

1. When discussing options for an electronic medical records system, the chief executive nurse asks you what cost of ownership is. What is your best response?
   A. Cost of ownership is the purchase price of an electronic medical records system.
   B. Cost of ownership is the total cost of using a good or service.
   C. Cost of ownership is the total cost of acquiring and using a good or service.
   D. Cost of ownership is the total cost of acquiring a good or service.

2. The chief nursing officer asks you what the common failures of procurement are. What is the best response?
   A. Clearly defining specifications
   B. Over- or understatement of work
   C. Poor planning in negotiations
   D. Detailing specifications

3. In planning for negotiations, the chief nursing officer asks you what is meant by negotiable factors. What is your best response?
   A. Negotiable factors are factors that will not stop the healthcare facility from agreeing with the vendor.
   B. Negotiable factors are factors that are nice to have but will not stop the healthcare facility from agreeing with the vendor.
   C. Negotiable factors are factors that must be in the agreement.
   D. Negotiable factors are factors agreed to with the vendor.

4. In preparations for negotiations, you ask the chief nursing officer to identify the breakpoint. She asks what is meant by the term *breakpoint*. What is your best response?
   A. Breakpoint is the least terms that are acceptable to the healthcare facility.
   B. Breakpoint is the best terms that are acceptable to the healthcare facility.
   C. Breakpoint is when the healthcare facility decides to settle with the vendor.
   D. Breakpoint is a cooling-off period when both parties break from negotiations.

5. **During your preparations for negotiations, you mention the term _bargaining range_. The chief nursing officer asks for you to explain this term. What is your best response?**

   A. The difference between the healthcare facility's initial offer and the healthcare facility's final offer is the bargaining range.

   B. The difference between the healthcare facility's counteroffer and the vendor's final offer is the bargaining range.

   C. The difference between the healthcare facility's initial offer and the vendor's counteroffer is the bargaining range.

   D. The difference between the healthcare facility's initial offer and the vendor's final offer is the bargaining range.

6. **During preparation for negotiations, the attorney mentions including a disincentive clause in the contract. After the meeting, the chief nursing officer asks you to give an example of a disincentive. What is your best response?**

   A. The healthcare facility will penalize the vendor 1% of the price for each month over the scheduled deadline.

   B. The healthcare facility will give the vendor 1% of the price for each month the system is delivered before the scheduled deadline.

   C. The healthcare facility will give the vendor 1% of the price for delivering the system on schedule.

   D. The healthcare facility will walk away from the contract.

7. **Throughout preparation for negotiations, the term _value_ has been discussed. The chief executive officer asks you to explain the meaning of value as related to negotiations. What is your best response?**

   A. Value is expected performance when the contract is executed.

   B. Value is the promise the vendor makes to the healthcare facility to deliver a product or service.

   C. Value is the perception of worth. The perception of value is used in negotiation to create a relatively low-cost incentive to reach the terms of a contract.

   D. Value is time spent negotiating with the vendor.

8. **During negotiations, the vendor requested progress payments. The chief nursing officer asks you to explain that term. What is the best response?**

   A. A progress payment is payment for noncapital expenses incurred by the vendor during the project.

   B. A progress payment is payment for capital expenses incurred by the vendor during the project.

   C. A progress payment is a payment for future work that the vendor will perform during the project.

   D. A progress payment is payment to the vendor for work completed during the project.

9. **In preparation for negotiations, the chief nursing officer was reading about good faith negotiations. She asks you to explain. What is the best response?**

   A. Negotiating in good faith means that a party is at the breakpoint.
   B. Negotiating in good faith means that a party is not sincerely interested in reaching an agreement.
   C. Negotiating in good faith means that a party is sincerely interested in reaching an agreement.
   D. Negotiating in good faith means that the vendor is at the breakpoint.

10. **During negotiations, the vendor proposes that disputes be handled by an arbitrator. The chief nursing officer asks you to explain the term. What is the best response?**

   A. An arbitrator meets with both parties to identify all the facts related to negotiations.
   B. An arbitrator meets with both parties to identify facts that are in dispute.
   C. An arbitrator unilaterally settles disputes.
   D. An arbitrator helps both parties settle a dispute.

CORRECT ANSWERS AND RATIONALES

1. C. Cost of ownership is the total cost of acquiring and using a good or service.
2. B. Over- or understatement of work
3. B. Negotiable factors are factors that are nice to have but will not stop the healthcare facility from agreeing with the vendor.
4. A. Breakpoint is the least terms that are acceptable to the healthcare facility.
5. C. The difference between the healthcare facility's initial offer and the vendor's counteroffer is the bargaining range.
6. A. The healthcare facility will penalize the vendor 1% of the price for each month over the scheduled deadline.
7. C. Value is the perception of worth. The perception of value is used in negotiation to create a relatively low-cost incentive to reach the terms of a contract.
8. C. A progress payment is a payment for future work that the vendor will perform during the project.
9. B. Negotiating in good faith means that a party is sincerely interested in reaching an agreement.
10. C. An arbitrator unilaterally settles disputes.

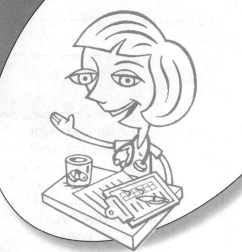

chapter 9

Clinical Disaster Recovery

LEARNING OBJECTIVES

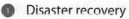

1. Disaster recovery
2. Risk assessment
3. Disaster recovery plan
4. Disaster recovery options
5. Disaster recovery operations

KEY TERMS

Business impact analysis	Indirect impact
Catastrophic event	Legacy system
Chain of command	Natural disasters
Classes of emergency	Outsourcing
Corrective measures	Point of failure
Data synchronization point	Preventive measures
Detective measures	Recovery point objective (RPO)
Direct impact	Recovery time objective (RTO)
Disaster	Risk
Disaster drills	Risk responses
Disaster recovery	Risk tolerance
Downtime procedures	Service level of agreement (SLA)
Emergency operations center (EOC)	Tier system
FUD factor	Unseen fail point
Human-made disaster	

1. Disaster Recovery

A **disaster** is a **catastrophic event** that may cause significant damage and possible loss of life. Catastrophic events include fire, floods, and powerful storms that place the ability to care for patients at **risk**. With conversion from paper to electronic medical records, a healthcare facility is exposed to being unable to access patient information and process medical orders during a power failure.

Let's say a wind storm causes a power disruption to the healthcare facility. The initial problem is administering medication. Some healthcare facilities use a computer on wheels (COW), which is a cart that contains a computer and medication for a group of patients. The computer is used to access the electronic medical records system (eMAR). Medication drawn on the COW are typically locked. Entering a code into the COW opens the drawer. The COW is powered by a rechargeable battery that has a limited life of maybe 4 hours. Drawers usually can also be opened with a key.

Electrical power is needed to power computers at the nurse's desk, recharge the COW, power the local area network, power the network server, power the application server where the eMAR program resides, and power the database server where patient information is stored (see Chapter 7). If one of those devices lacks power, then the nurse is unable to access the eMAR that contains information needed to administer medication to patients.

A disaster can have significant impact on the healthcare facility other than loss of power. For example, staffing is a critical issue. Are staff members able to come to the hospital during a disaster? Roads may be closed, staff members may experience personal disasters at home, and staff members may simply prefer to stay home rather than risk getting injured on the way to work. The administration may be able to hold over the current shift; however, at some point, the current staff needs a break. No staff can work more than 16 hours in a row. As a result, the healthcare facility will lack staff to care for patients.

Another concern is supplies. Food, linens, medications, and other material needed to care for patients may not be refurnished because vendors are unable to deliver goods to the healthcare facility. The longer the impact of the disaster, the higher the risk the healthcare facility is unable to care for patients.

A disaster can also include failure of heating, ventilation, and air conditioning or loss of key employees because of injury on or off the job or if they are called up for military service. A staff or vendor strike of the healthcare facility can place the healthcare facility in disaster mode.

> ### NURSING ALERT
>
> Anything that can arise fear, uncertainty, or doubt of continuity can lead to a disaster. This is commonly referred to as the **FUD factor**.

Categorizing a Disaster

A disaster can be categorized in a number of ways. These include general classifications. There are two general classifications of disasters. These are:

- **Natural disasters**: A natural disaster is an act of nature such as storms, floods, and earthquakes. Natural disasters cannot be prevented.

- **Human-made disaster**: A human-made disaster is an act of humans such as failure of the infrastructure or a hazardous material spill. A human-made disaster may be preventable by monitoring and implementing procedures that reduce the likelihood of such an event.

Each of these classifications can be further categorized as a **class of emergency**. A class of emergency defines the emergency condition by the length of time of the emergency. Classes are:

- Class 1: Class 1 is an emergency that lasts a few hours such as a brief power outage or an injury onsite.
- Class 2: Class 2 is an emergency that lasts 72 hours or less and is less serious than a Class 1 emergency such as a contained fire that causes slight damage to the healthcare facility.
- Class 3: Class 3 is an emergency that lasts more than 72 hours that affects one area of the healthcare facility such as the data center.
- Class 4: Class 4 is an emergency that last more than 72 hours that affects the entire healthcare facility.
- Class 5: Class 5 is an emergency that affects the entire community such a storm or flooding.

An alternative classification method is the **tier system**. The tier system separates operational functions into three tiers. These are:

- Tier 1: Tier 1 consists of functions that need to be operational with the first 72 hours of the disaster.
- Tier 2: Tier 2 consists of functions that need to be operational by the end of the first week of the disaster.
- Tier 3: Tier 3 consists of functions that need to be operational by the end of the first month of the disaster.

NURSING ALERT

All healthcare facilities are prone to internal and external cyber attacks (see Chapter 10).

2. Risk Assessment

A risk is the possibility of harm or long-term loss as a result of an event. Risk assessment is a process for assessing the magnitude of the potential loss related to interruption of operations if such a disaster occurs. **Risk tolerance** is the acceptance of risk by the organization with little or no effort to mitigate or avoid the risk. The reaction of an organization to risk is called the **risk response**.

The most obvious risk is loss of life related directly or indirectly to the disaster. **Direct impact** occurs if the wind causes a tree to fall on a patient who is outside the healthcare facility. **Indirect impact** occurs when the patient is unable to receive proper medication because the nurse is unable to access the electronic medical system because of a power outage related to storm damage.

Three questions should be asked when performing a risk assessment. These are:

- What is the risk?
- What is the probability that the risky event will occur?
- What is the impact to the healthcare facility should the risky event occur?

The risk assessment must consider direct and indirect impact on the healthcare facility. In addition to functional operating losses such as loss of patient information and disruptions to the healthcare facility's network in a power failure, secondary losses must also be considered. A secondary loss is a consequence that may occur as results of the disaster such as HIPAA (Health Insurance Portability and Accountability Act) violations, financial losses, and litigation.

Systematically examine events that could harm the healthcare facility. Assess if sufficient precautions have been taken to protect the healthcare facility from those events. Identify mission critical functions and evaluate contingency plans in case critical functions are disrupted.

NURSING ALERT

Do not overlook the environment such as drinking water, power, and heat.

HIPAA requires that a risk assessment be performed as part of the healthcare facility's **disaster recovery** plan. All assets must be reviewed and vulnerabilities identified. The focus of a HIPAA risk assessment is on data security and the potential effects of the event.

Table 9–1 lists departments within the healthcare facility that should be assessed when performing a risk assessment. Each department is critical to the successful operation of the healthcare facility.

TABLE 9–1 Departments within the Healthcare Facility that Should Be Assessed

Patient care services	Pharmacy	Laboratory
Management information systems	Dietary	Patient billing and coding
Order processing	Human resources	Payroll
Imaging	Respiratory therapy	Facilities services
Materials management	Shipping and receiving	Finance
Clinics	Patient registration	Administrative support
Security	Patient access	Case management

Business Impact Analysis

A **business impact analysis** focuses on the impact the disaster has on the operations of the healthcare facility. The initial steps in a business impact analysis are to identify and prioritize applications and data that are required for the organization to function and the impact on the operations of the organization that may occur if those application and data were not available.

A healthcare facility may have many applications and many databases. However, to assess the impact of each requires that the nurse informatics specialist reviews each in detail. The challenge is that detailed information about older systems may not be readily available. Furthermore, there is limited detail available about newer application because details are considered by many vendors as proprietary information and not shared with customers.

Here are steps that should be included in the business impact analysis:

- Assess the minimum effort needed to maintain operational levels of the healthcare facility.
- Review the impact of disruptions on patient care units.
- Identify steps in all processes.
- Estimate recovery point objectives (see Recovery Point Objectives) for each patient care unit.
- Assess the needs of direct support departments such as the pharmacy and laboratory.
- Identify gaps in the operations that can fail.

NURSING ALERT

Always keep in mind who is affected by the disaster. These include patients, patients' families, employees, employees' families, vendors, government agencies, regulatory authorities, the community at large, and the news media.

Legacy Systems

A **legacy system** is a process critical to the operations of the healthcare facility that has not been reviewed or upgraded for a long time. A legacy system can be a computer-based system, manual system, or a combination. The system may be totally under the control of the healthcare facility or provided by a vendor. Common to all legacy systems is that the system has been operating without problems for many years, so much so in fact that managers tend to not manage the system. In essence, managers forget about legacy systems.

Legacy systems become problematic when the system ceases to operate such as during a disaster. No one presently on staff is familiar with the details of the system, especially the computerized portions of the system. The vendor may no longer be in business. No one is available to fix the legacy system on short notice—if at all. The staff that is intimately knowledgeable about the system has long retired.

Therefore, it is critical during a risk assessment to identify legacy systems and prepare to provide adequate support for that system or replace legacy system with a system that can be supported by the present staff.

Points of Failure

The initial step in the risk assessment is to identify points of failure within the healthcare facility. A **point of failure** is an element in the healthcare facility's operation that might fail such as failure of the local area network from transmitting electronic data throughout the facility.

Identify points of failure by conducting an information technology (IT) audit for all processes. Begin with the end point and then follow the process to the source. Each step in the process is a point of failure. That is, the process fails if the step cannot be performed.

Let's say you are auditing the eMAR system. The end point is when the nurse is using eMAR to know what medications is to be given to a patient; the source is the database that is used to store the patient's medication record. The process includes:

- The nurse logging on to the computer, network, and the eMAR application
- The computer connecting to the network and the network transmits patient medication records
- The eMAR application running and connected to the network
- The database that contains the patient medication records operating and connecting the database
- Patient information being available in the database

Following the process to identify points of failure also requires tracing the hardware used to access the information. Hardware includes computers, cables, servers, and other computing devices. A good approach to use is to follow the cable. With the assistance of a management information systems (MIS) technician, start at the network cable leading from the computer or the Wi-Fi connection (see Chapter 7) used by the COW. A network cable usually leads into the wall or the ceiling and ends in a communication closet located somewhere in the hallway. If Wi-Fi is used, there is a Wi-Fi transceiver (sends and receives signals) in the vicinity of the COW. The Wi-Fi transceiver is connected by a network cable to the communication closet.

The communication closet is the location where cables from nearby networking devices converge into a single connection to the data center. The data center is the central location where data, databases, and servers reside. It is important to ask the MIS technician to walk you through the trail from the computer to the data. Take note of each hardware component. Each is a point of failure and could disrupt the nurse from administering medications to the patient.

Recovery Point Objective

A **recovery point objective (RPO)** is the acceptable period of time when a process can be unavailable. Let's return to the process of administering medication to patients. The RPO for the medication administration process is different depending on the unit within the healthcare facility and the patient's condition.

For example, a patient is in crisis such as one in the emergency department or in a critical care unit requires medication immediately. The RPO is zero. Nurses must be able to administer medication when the medication becomes available. After a patient is stabilized and moved to an acute unit, medication is administered on a schedule expected in extreme situations when the patient receives a start medication. Let's assume that medication is scheduled every 3 hours. The RPO can be 3 hours, assuming the downtime begins immediately after the scheduled medication is administered.

Knowing the RPO for each step in a process enables the nurse informatics specialist to develop a disaster recovery plan that identifies the potential impact of a point of failure and devise a plan of action to restore functionality during the failure.

Recovery Time Objective

The **recovery time objective (RTO)** is the time needed by MIS to restore the process when a failure occurs. This differs from the RPO in that the RPO is determined by the business process, and the RTO is determined by the MIS recovery process and assessed by the MIS department.

Both the RPO and RTO must be determined as part of the disaster recovery plan so that designers of the plan can develop contingencies to keep patient care at an acceptable level during the disaster.

Data Synchronization Point

Data recovery is a critical element of every disaster recovery plan. Data recovery is the process of restoring data after an event that disabled the database. A database contains patient medical records. A disaster recovery plan typically contains a process that restores the database from a backed up version of the database. A database backup is a copy of the database that is copied to the primary database to restore the database to a state before the failure.

The nurse informatics specialist must identify the **data synchronization point** when developing the disaster recovery. The data synchronization point is when data is backed up. Depending on the design of the application, data can be backed up either immediately after a transaction (see Chapter 4) or on a schedule.

A transaction is the insertion of data after a clinical event such as updates to the patient's medical records or documenting that the patient received medication. After data is inserted into the database, the data is automatically copied to other databases, commonly referred to a mirrored database. The mirrored database and the primary database are synchronized. That is, the latest data is stored in both databases. The data synchronization point is relatively immediate.

A scheduled database backup occurs on prescribed periods such as every 2 hours, every 8 hours, or every 12 hours. These are data synchronization points. Data entered into the primary database between data synchronization points is lost. Restored data reflects data stored at the data synchronization point.

Knowing the data synchronization point enables the nurse informatics specialist to develop a contingency plan for failures that occur between data synchronization points.

NURSING ALERT

Regulatory agencies required healthcare MIS executives to identify critical systems and develop plans to recover when confronted with a disaster.

Unseen Fail Points

An **unseen fail point** is an element in the process that is not obvious to the nurse informatics specialist during the disaster recovery survey process. Most of these are software elements that are necessary to restore functionality to the computing device.

Computing devices require an operating system (see Chapter 1). The operating system is usually configured for the computing device and the needs of the healthcare facility. The computing device runs an application such as the eMAR that interfaces over the network with the database server that stores patients' health records.

If the computing device fails, technicians must install the operating system, configure the operating system, and install the application onto the computing device. The unseen fail points are instructions on how to do this and a list of the configurations. Let's say that the disaster occurred at 2 am. Will the technicians on site be able to restore the functionality even though installations and configurations may rarely be performed on that shift? Although more knowledgeable technicians might be on call at home, a communication connection at the data center, at the technician's home, or at both may be down.

The nurse informatics specialist who conducts the disaster recovery audit must consider the unseen fail points. The challenge is to recognize those fail points, especially because the nurse informatics specialist may not be familiar with the subtleties of the technology. The best approach is to work with the MIS department and ask them questions about the processes. Do not make assumptions. If the MIS department says, "We'll reload the application," be sure to ask where the application is (e.g., on CD, downloaded from the vendor's website). Follow the thought process by asking:

- Who installs the application?
- Has that person installed the application in the past?
- Are there special configurations that need to be made to the application?
- Are there written instructions on how to install and configure the application?
- Where are those instructions stored?
- Does the person who is installing the application know where to access the instructions?

There can be an endless number of questions to ask, but it is important that you know exactly how the restore is performed. The answers to your questions may expose a weakness in the planned recovery process. For example, the technician may not know where the instructions are located to restore the application. The technician may be counting on calling the on-call technician for help, not realizing that the communication connection may be unavailable.

NURSING ALERT

Data centers may use an automatic process to reinstall application and restore function after a disaster. The automatic process is driven by a script written by a technician that executes all steps in the process. The technician on duty still must know how to run the automatic process.

3. Disaster Recovery Plan

Disaster recovery is the process of restoring function to the healthcare facility during and after the disaster. Critical to the recovery is the disaster recovery plan. A disaster recovery plan contains processes to follow for specific disasters and is a component of a broad plan called a business continuity plan.

The objective of disaster recovery is to return the healthcare facility to normal operational levels. Achieving normal operational levels can be gradual with high-priority items returning first or immediately. The return to normal operational levels depends on the nature of the disaster and the effort required to restore operations.

Let's say a severe storm made it impossible for staff to arrive for their shift. Administrative staff members who are on site can be recruited to perform non–licensed-required duties such as transporting food from the kitchen to the floors. Food service might be slow, but food will arrive, and the patients will be fed. As the storm subsides and staff arrives, food service returns to normal operations.

Disaster Recovery versus Business Continuity

The disaster recovery plan focuses on returning the healthcare facility to marginal functionality within the first week of the disaster. This is like picking up the pieces and restoring some semblance of order from a chaotic situation. A business continuity plan is focused on the long term restoration of healthcare operations beyond 1 week after the disaster.

Let's say a storm disrupted power to the healthcare facility. The disaster recovery plan focuses on using battery backup power and the healthcare facility's own generator to provide power to keep the healthcare facility marginally operational. The business continuity plan focuses on how to reduce the likelihood of the power disruption occurring in the future.

Elements of a Disaster Recovery Plan

In addition to providing a roadmap to restore functionality to the healthcare facility, a disaster recovery plan also defines control measures. A disaster recovery control measure is a process for dealing with an element of a disaster. There are three elements of a disaster specified in a disaster recovery plan. These are:

- **Preventive measures**: Preventive measures are processes that prevent a disaster from occurring. For example, placing power lines underground prevents loss of power caused by a storm disrupting power lines.

- **Detective measures**: Detective measures are processes that discover that a disaster has occurred. For example, activation of a fire alarm signals a fire is a detective measure common to all healthcare facilities.
- **Corrective measures**: Corrective measures are processes that restore function to the healthcare facility during or after a disaster. For example, an electrical generator provides power to the healthcare facility until the main power is restored.

Assumptions

A disaster recovery plan is based on assumptions of what disaster is probable. It is important that potential disasters be listed in the disaster recovery plan. A list of assumptions should be listed for each potential disaster. The assumption should focus on the probability of the disaster's occurring supported by evidence.

For example, there might be small tremors over the years but no earthquake sufficient to cause structural damage based on a review of 100 years of data for the area. The assumption is that there will never be a significant earthquake, and therefore there is no need to include an earthquake in the disaster recovery plan.

It goes without saying that assumptions are sometimes not true. That is, an earthquake can happen, and the healthcare facility will be unprepared to recover from the earthquake. It is therefore critical that a disaster recovery plan considers all types of disasters even though a certain disaster maybe remotely based on history.

Risk Tolerance

The level of detail addressed in the disaster recovery plan is driven by regulatory compliance and by the amount of risk administrators will tolerate. For example, during normal operations, an administrator may staff at 110% required staffing levels, anticipating that 10% of the staff will not show for work for various reasons. The administrator is willing to spend 10% in compensation that is needed to protect against a staff shortage. That is, if everyone shows for work, 10% of the staff will have nothing to do but will be paid. The administrator is willing to take that risk. However, the administrator is not willing to staff at 100% and take the risk that 10% of the staff will not show for work, which results in a staffing level of 90%.

Each risk identified in the risk assessment is considered when developing the disaster recovery plan. Administrators must decide a response for each risk. Responses are to:

- Accept: Accept the risk and deal with it if the risk materializes.
- Mitigate: Reduce the risk by doing something that lowers the probability that the risk will occur.
- Transfer: Transfer the risk to a vendor. The vendor takes on the responsibility of deciding how to respond to the risk. The healthcare facility is still exposed to the risk, but the response to the risk is transferred to the vendor.
- Avoid: The administrator can change the situation to avoid the risk entirely.

Deciding on a response to a risk is not easy because the administrator must balance the effort to respond to the risk with the likelihood that the risk will materialize. The response will likely cost money except if the administrator accepts the risk. The administrator must determine if the response is worth the expenditure.

Low-Level Focus

The disaster recovery plan must focus on details of the operation and provide a solution for dealing with expected and unexpected situations that may arise. Here are common details that should be considered in a disaster recovery plan.

- What is the staffing level needed to maintain minimal functionality?
- Are staffing levels maintained at the minimal level for all shifts?
- How will staff arrive during a disaster?
- Where will staff be stationed in the healthcare facility during a disaster?
- Does the staff have the skillsets necessary to provide minimal functionality?
- If there is one chef and the replacement chef is unable to report for more than 16 hours, then who is going to prepare meals for the patients and staff?
- Where will off-duty staff, who are not leaving the facility go to sleep, shower, and change clothes?
- Is sufficient food available for patients and staff for the duration of the disaster and the first week after the disaster?
- Will employees be more concerned about the disaster affecting their families at home than coming to work?
- Are employees able to come to work if mass transit is not operational?
- How long will supplies last (e.g., medications, food, linens)?

> ### NURSING ALERT
>
> Do not overlook how staff will communicate with each other during a disaster. Telephone communication within and external to the facility may be unavailable.

4. Disaster Recovery Options

There are many options to recover from a disaster, each requiring that preparation be made in advance to ensure that the recovery option is available at the time of the disaster. Key to recovery is restoring MIS functionality to the healthcare facility. MIS functionality includes applications, databases, servers, the network, and computing devices used by the staff to care for patients.

In an ideal world, the healthcare facility has a fully operational data center at a remote location that can be immediately connected to the healthcare facility during or shortly after a disaster. This is referred to as a hot site because the site is fully operational and has all applications, databases, and computing devices as found in the healthcare facility's primary site.

A less costly option is called a warm site. A warm site is a remote location that can be prepared to act as a data center for the facility within a week or so. Applications, databases, and servers may have to be configured.

The least costly and one that requires the most lead time is referred to as a cold site. A cold site has no equipment. The equipment must be installed and configured, taking a month or so before the cold site can become operational.

An alternative to the healthcare facility's operating a data center is for the healthcare facility to outsource the data center to a vendor. **Outsourcing** is a way to offload the risk associated with running a data center. That is, the vendor takes on the responsibility of providing disaster recovery processes if the data center becomes involved in a disaster. Outsourcing also enables the healthcare facility to respond to changes in capacity. As demand increases, the healthcare facility acquires new capacity by outsourcing services. Likewise, outsourcing services can be terminated as demand decreases.

Outsourcing data centers must be HIPAA security compliant. Key to compliance is policies and controls. Policies of the outsourcing organization must reflect HIPAA requirements. These policies must be enforced by controls embedded into applications. For example, a requirement is for access to be limited according to the need to know. Controls are security groups. Each group is defined by function, and access to systems is granted based on the needs of each group. An employee is assigned to a security group based on the employee's position in the healthcare facility.

A data center must be in a low-risk area to natural disasters such as floods, hurricanes, tornadoes, and earthquakes. Likewise, employees of the outsourcing data center must live in low-risk areas too. A data center's service to the healthcare facility is dependent on its employees. If employees are personally affected by the disaster, then there is a high risk that the data center is unable to provide service.

The data center, whether or not the data center is outsourced, must have physical controls to access the facility (see Chapter 10). These include video monitoring, biometrics access (e.g., fingerprinting), computing devices placed with internal secured areas (e.g., cages), and security personnel throughout the facility 24 hours a day, 7 days a week.

The data center must have a high level of redundancy. If any element of the data center fails, two or three elements can take its place quickly. For example, if a database server fails, a replacement can be fully operational within an hour.

A backup power source is necessary for all healthcare facilities. There are two types of backup power sources. These are battery backup and an onsite generator. The battery backup is used to power certain electrical devices such as computing devices for a few hours. The onsite generator is used to power certain electrical devices until the main power source is back on line (see Chapter 10). Only electrical devices that are needed for patient care should be on the backup power system because limited power may be available during the disaster.

Employees of the outsourcing firm must be trained in the Electronic Protected Health Information (ePHI) as set forth in HIPAA (see Chapter 10).

> **NURSING ALERT**
>
> Make sure that backup power sources are always in working condition and are sufficient to meet the current needs of the healthcare facility. More backup power is required as healthcare facilities implement electronic systems.

Service Level of Agreement

Outsourcing transfers the healthcare facility's responsibility to provide the outsourcing service to a vendor. It is important to understand that the healthcare facility remains responsible for the service, although the contract with the vendor appears to transfer those responsibilities to the vendor (see Chapter 8). That is, failure of the vendor to provide the service on behalf of the healthcare facility does not relieve the healthcare facility from the responsibility of providing the service to patients.

The vendor must provide the healthcare facility with a **service level of agreement (SLA)**. An SLA contains objective metrics that both the vendor and the healthcare facility can use to measure the vendor's performance. The SLA is typically part of the contract with the vendor and contains remedies if the vendor fails to perform to the expectations of the SLA (see Chapter 8).

The SLA specifies the minimum service that the healthcare facility will receive from the vendor. Metrics used to measure the service depend on the nature of the service. Let's say the vendor provides data center services. A common metric to use is mean time to recovery (MTTR). MTTR is the average time necessary to restore the data center functionality to the healthcare facility.

If the vendor manufactures computing devices such as a server, the commonly used metric is mean time between failures (MTBF). MTBF is the average time period that the computing device will work before the device breaks down. This is important to know when acquiring and managing computing devices. Manufacturers test computing devices under various conditions and simulate extended usages. Test results identify a time range after which the computing device is likely to fail. You should acquire the computing device that meets your specifications and has the longest MTBF.

Here are other commonly used metrics:

- Turnaround time (TAT): TAT is the time that is necessary to complete a specific task.

- Uptime (UT): UT is the amount of time that the application, computing device, or data center is functioning. For example, a computing device maybe unavailable for 4 hours a week while the MIS department performs maintenance on the device.

- First call resolution (FCR): FCR is a percentage of calls to a helpdesk that are resolved without the callers calling the helpdesk again.

- Time service factor (TSF): TSF is a percentage of calls that are asked within a specific time period.

- Abandonment rate (ABA): ABA is the percentage of callers whose calls are not answered. The caller who is on a wait queue hangs up.

- Average speed to answer (ASA): ASA is the number of seconds needed for the helpdesk to answer the phone.

NURSING ALERT

Keep a log of how long each computing device is operating. Consider replacing the device when the device usage is close to the time when the device might fail. Anticipating failure ensures that the computing device is always available.

The MIS department and operating units of the healthcare facility should have an operational level of agreement. An operational level of agreement is similar in concept to the SLA except the agreement is between internal entities within the healthcare facility. For example, the MIS department agrees to respond to a nurse's problem with the electronic medication administration records system within a half hour of a call to the help desk. The response is material and not simply an MIS department representative answering the telephone. That is, someone knowledgeable about the system will address the nurse's concerns. MIS managers can staff and plan according to the operational level agreement.

Both SLA and an operational level of agreement focus on outcomes and not how those outcomes are achieved except that methodologies will comply with regulatory requirements. That is, the vendor or MIS may bring in another source to meet the obligation to deliver the outcome.

5. Disaster Recovery Operations

The healthcare facility is required to create a hospital emergency incident command system (HEICS) that takes over operations of the healthcare facility during a disaster or emergency. HEICS has a **chain of command** that enables fast, ongoing assessment of the disaster and the impact the disaster has on the healthcare facility's operations. The HEICS structure enables the emergency incident response team to respond to known problems and anticipate and mitigate problems that might be forthcoming.

The chain of command structure is documented in a Job Action Sheet. The Job Action Sheet lists each position in the command structure and the corresponding roles and responsibilities. The Job Action Sheet and all information about the disaster are shared in the emergency incident command site. Each member of the emergency response team can view, assess, and determine the course of action appropriate to the team member's responsibility.

Four Sections of the Chain of Command

The emergency response is led by the emergency incident commander (IC). The emergency IC is the person in charge of the emergency response. All decisions rest with that person, although the emergency IC relies heavily on subject matter experts such as the medical team and governmental emergency management.

There are four areas of concern for the emergency IC and the healthcare facility's administrators. Each area is called a section and has a section chief who is responsible for addressing issues within the domain of that section. Sections are:

- Operations: Operations involves maintaining an adequate level of patient care. These include not only medical care, but also food service and housekeeping.

- Logistics: Logistics is the management of resources, both internal and external to the healthcare facility. Logistics involve staffing, medical supplies, food supplies, both receiving and distribution within the facility, and garbage removal—everything necessary for caring for patients and the staff during the disaster.

- Planning: Planning involves the emergency response team anticipating needs and devising a way to meet those needs in advance. This includes developing a disaster recovery plan.

- Finance: The healthcare facility must have funds to pay for ongoing operations and for expenditures that are associated with responding to the emergency such as overtime cost. Furthermore, the healthcare facility must ensure that incoming revenue stream is not disrupted. For example, patients will postpone selected care until the healthcare facility has recovered from the disaster; therefore, anticipated revenues from those procedures will not be realized.

NURSING ALERT

Keep a copy of the contact information for all employees off site. This enables the disaster recovery team to contact employees from anywhere during a disaster. Highlight employees who are critical to the operations.

Emergency Operations Center

The **emergency operations center (EOC)** is a location in the healthcare facility where the disaster is managed. Typically, the EOC is located in a central location within the facility such as a large conference room or auditorium.

The room should be divided into five areas. One area is for the emergency IC, and each of the other four are for a section. Each section must be clearly identified and always staffed by at least one representative of that section's team. Communication connections should be established for each area, enabling free flow of communication to the field, if necessary.

The emergency IC section should display the Job Action Sheet on a white board or flip chart so each member of the emergency response team can clearly identify their roles. Another board or flip chart should list the status of operations, preferably by unit and department. The status should include required staffing levels, actual staffing levels, supplies, and other factors required to operate the healthcare facility.

The status should be projected per shift per day for the entire week. A shift is the work day for employees. For example, some nurses work 12-hour shifts, others work 8-hour shifts. The status helps each section chief anticipate problems in the near future.

> **NURSING ALERT**
>
> The Joint Commission (formerly the Joint Commission on Accreditation of Healthcare Organizations [JCAHO]) requires every hospital to have a hospital emergency incident command system. The Joint Commission has no enforcement powers; however, regulatory agencies that have enforcement powers and third-party payers look at The Joint Commission rating as a guide to determine if the healthcare facility is meeting industry standards. HIPAA requires that a disaster recovery plan exists for every healthcare facility.

Downtime Procedures

Downtime procedures are processes that are enacted when a disaster or emergency occurs. These are well-thought-through steps that, if followed, will maintain the functionality of the healthcare facility. There are two elements of a downtime procedure. These are to keep the healthcare facility operational and to recover after the disaster has passed.

For example, nurses and practitioners need to document assessments in the patient's medical record. Before the disaster, assessments were recorded in the eMAR. However, the eMAR is unavailable because of a power outage. Therefore, assessments are recorded on paper as part of the downtime procedure. When the disaster is over, a procedure is necessary to record those assessments in the eMAR; otherwise, the electronic medical record is incomplete.

All downtime procedures should be incorporated in the disaster recovery plan.

> **NURSING ALERT**
>
> Make sure employees who evacuate the premises take their belongings with them. They will not be able to go home without their car keys, house keys, and other personal belongings.

Disaster Drills

The healthcare facility must hold **disaster drills** on a regular schedule during the course of the year. Disaster drills should simulate real-life disasters to test the response of the emergency response team. Although drills are scheduled, the drill should be held spontaneously. The emergency response team and the facility staff should not be alerted about the drill because disasters are rarely known in advance.

The disaster drill can be segmented. For example, the data center or a portion of the data center can operate on backup power for a few hours to test whether or not the backup power is sufficient to support the data center.

Backup activities are tested during a disaster drill to ensure that expected operational function is maintained by using the backup. The disaster recovery plan must be modified if backup activities are unable to support operational levels.

Here are factors to consider when planning a disaster drill:

- All employees, including administrators, must participate in the disaster drill.

- All employees should perform their expected roles in a disaster during the disaster drill.

- Be sure that the disaster drill is realistic. A real disaster increases stress on staff. You should assess how well the staff will perform under the stress of a disaster.

- Include community services such as police and fire personnel in the disaster drill.

- The goal is to find weaknesses in the disaster response and not simply walk through tasks associated with the disaster drill.

- Make sure staff are trained to perform roles secondary to their primary responsibility (e.g., administrators are able to move food carts from the kitchen to the floors).

NURSING ALERT

A disaster recovery plan that is untested regularly should not be considered a valid disaster recovery plan because the disaster recovery plan has not been validated by scheduled testing.

CASE STUDY

CASE 1

As the nurse informatics specialists for a 1-unit healthcare facility, you are asked to devise a disaster recovery process for the new electronic medical administration records (eMAR) system. Practitioners write medication orders either on paper or in the computerized practitioner order entry system (CPOE). Paper medication orders are faxed to the pharmacy. CPOE orders are electronically sent to the pharmacy. The pharmacy takes the order and enters the order in the eMAR. The eMAR entry is compared against the original order by the nurse, the nurse activates the order on the eMAR, and the medication is ready to be administered per the order. The nurse displays the patient's eMAR on the computer and administers the medication based on entries in the eMAR. The nurse also uses the eMAR to document that the medication was administered to the patient according the practitioner's order. There is no paper medical administration record documentation available on the unit. The executive nurse and the administration have concerns about how medication will be administered during a power outage. Specifically, they have the following questions. What are your best responses?

QUESTION 1. How practitioners write new medication orders when the CPOE system is unavailable?
ANSWER: Each unit will have a supply of blank paper orders. Practitioners can write new orders on the blank paper order or call a telephone order into the unit. The nurse then writes the order on the blank paper order sheet. A staff member will then walk medication orders to the pharmacy for processing and return to the unit with the medication.

QUESTION 2. How will nurses receive a copy of the eMAR during a power outage?
ANSWER: There will be several computers on selected units plugged into the backup power supply. Each of these computers will be directly attached to a printer. The printer will also be plugged into the backup power supply. Every 4 hours and every 2 hour for critical care units, a printable version of all eMARs will be sent to these selected computers. Nurses from each unit will print the unit's eMAR from the selected computer at the first sign of a power outage.

QUESTION 3. What will happen if the power outage lasts more than 24 hours?
ANSWER: The printed MAR will be sufficient to record medication administration for 24 hours. After 24 hours, nurses will create a new paper medication records using a blank MAR that will be supplied to the units. Nurses will base the new MAR on the temporary print MAR and medication orders in the patient's chart.

QUESTION 4. When power is restored, the eMAR system will not reflect medication administered during the power outage. How should this be resolved?

ANSWER: The paper MAR forms used during the power outage will be placed in the patient's chart. The nurse will indicate in the eMAR that specific medications were administered during the power outage and documented on paper in the patient's chart. Anyone reading the eMAR will then know to refer to the paper chart to see medication administered during the power outage.

FINAL CHECK-UP

1. **The executive nurse is reviewing the disaster recovery plan and asks the nurse informatics specialist to explain the difference between a natural disaster and a human-made disaster. What is the best response?**

   A. A natural disaster is caused by an accident. A human-made disaster is caused by an unintentional or intentional act of a person.

   B. A natural disaster is caused by an act of nature. A human-made disaster is caused by an unintentional or intentional act of a person.

   C. A natural disaster is caused by an act of nature. A human-made disaster is caused by not preparing for the natural disaster.

   D. A natural disaster is caused by a preventable act of nature. A human-made disaster is caused by an unintentional or intentional act of a person.

2. **The nurse executive asks you to explain the difference between a disaster recovery plan and a business continuity plan. What is your best response?**

   A. A disaster recovery plan focuses on restoring operations. Healthcare facilities do not have a business continuity plan because the healthcare facility is not a business.

   B. A disaster recovery plan focuses on restoring clinical operations. A business continuity plan focuses on restoring business operations.

   C. A disaster recovery plan focuses on restoring operations during the first week of the disaster. A business continuity plan focuses on restoring operations after the first week of the disaster.

   D. A disaster recovery plan focuses on restoring both clinical and business operations. A business continuity plan is not needed for a healthcare facility.

3. **The director of nursing is confused by the term *legacy system*. What is the best response?**

    A. A legacy system is a process that has not been reviewed or upgraded for a long time but provides an important process in the operations of the healthcare facility.

    B. A legacy system is a system provided by a vendor.

    C. A legacy system is an older version of the current system that is important to the operations of healthcare facility.

    D. A legacy system is the new version of a system that is important to the operations of the healthcare facility.

4. **The executive nurse is confused by the term *recovery point objective*. What is the best reply?**

    A. A recovery point objective is the acceptable period of time when a process can be unavailable.

    B. A recovery point objective is the acceptable period of time when a process can be available.

    C. A recovery point objective is the unacceptable period of time when a process can be unavailable.

    D. A recovery point objective is the unacceptable period of time when a process can be available.

5. **There seems to be confusion over the term *data synchronization point*. The executive nurse and the MIS director differ on the meaning of the term. What is the explanation of this term?**

    A. The data synchronization point is when data is used by the MIS department.

    B. The data synchronization point is when data is used by end users.

    C. The data synchronization point is when data is restored.

    D. The data synchronization point is when data is backed up.

6. **The executive nurse is reading about detective measures in the disaster recovery plan. She asks for an explanation. What is the best response?**

    A. Detective measures are processes that focus on the occurrence of the disaster.

    B. Detective measures are processes that prevent a disaster from occurring.

    C. Detective measures are processes that restore function to the healthcare facility during or after a disaster.

    D. Detective measures are processes that discover that a disaster occurred.

7. **The director of nursing asks you what options are available to respond to a risk. What is the best response?**

    A. Accept, mitigate, transfer, and avoid

    B. Accept, mitigate, and avoid

    C. Accept, transfer, and avoid

    D. Accept, mitigate, transfer, submit, and avoid

8. **The executive nurse was asked by the MIS director for her risk tolerance regarding risks associated with a disaster. The executive nurse asked you to explain the term *risk tolerance*. What is the best response?**

A. Risk tolerance is a measurement of how often a computing device will fail.

B. Risk tolerance is a response to risk.

C. Risk tolerance is an acceptable amount of risk by the administrator.

D. Risk tolerance is a measurement of how long a computing device can operate before the computing device fails.

9. **The MIS department's proposed disaster recovery plan speaks about a service level of agreement. The executive nurse asks you to explain this term. What is the best response?**

A. A service level of agreement is a contract that specifies the maximum level of service that a vendor will provide to the healthcare facility.

B. A service level of agreement is a contract that specifies the minimal level of service that a vendor will provide to the healthcare facility.

C. A service level of agreement is an understanding that specifies the minimal level of service that a vendor will provide to the healthcare facility.

D. A service level of agreement is an understanding that specifies the maximum level of service that a vendor will provide to the healthcare facility.

10. **The executive nurse asks you who is in charge during a disaster. What is the best response?**

A. Each unit manager

B. The president of the healthcare facility

C. The chief operating officer of the healthcare facility

D. The emergency incident commander

CORRECT ANSWERS AND RATIONALES

1. B. A natural disaster is caused by an act of nature. A human-made disaster is caused by an unintentional or intentional act of a person.
2. C. A disaster recovery plan focuses on restoring operations during the first week of the disaster. A business continuity plan focuses on restoring operations after the first week of the disaster.
3. A. A legacy system is a process that has not been reviewed or upgraded for a long time but provides an important process in the operations of the healthcare facility.
4. A. A recovery point objective is the acceptable period of time when a process can be unavailable.
5. D. The data synchronization point is when data is backed up.

6. D. Detective measures are processes that discover that a disaster occurred.
7. A. Accept, mitigates, transfer, and avoid.
8. C. Risk tolerance is an acceptable amount of risk by the administrator.
9. B. A service level of agreement is a contract that specifies the minimal level of service that a vendor will provide to the healthcare facility.
10. D. The emergency incident commander

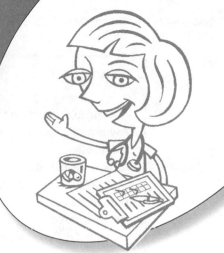

chapter 10

Clinical Systems Security

LEARNING OBJECTIVES

1. Security audit
2. HIPAA and HITECH Act
3. Proxy servers
4. Firewall
5. Encryption
6. Security on a wireless network
7. Spam
8. Denial of service attack
9. Identity theft
10. Computer viruses

KEY TERMS

Advanced Encryption Standard (AES)	Health Insurance Portability and
Asymmetric key encryption	Accountability Act (HIPAA)
Bluetooth	Information disclosure
Business associates	Omnibus rule
Cyclic redundancy check (CRC)	Packet filtering
Data at rest	Physical access
Data disposed	Protected health identifiers (PHIs)
Data encryption standard (DES)	Public key
Data in motion	Rootkit
Data in use	Secure Socket Link (SSL)
Database access points	Stateful inspection
Demilitarized zone (DMZ)	Symmetric key encryption
Digital certificates	Transport layer security (TLS)
Disabling services	Trojan horse
Health Information Technology for	Unauthorized access
Economic and Clinical Health	Wi-Fi
(HITECH) Act	Worms

Clinical systems security is a critical factor in providing healthcare because practitioners and other clinicians make treatment decisions that prevent or reverse life-threatening illness. Initially, the patient presents with a medical problem. The practitioner asks questions and performs a physical assessment. The practitioner then reviews the patient's medical records that include medications, test results, and other pertinent information that helps the practitioner decide the course of treatment. The practitioner trusts that the patient's medical records are intact and accurate and contain information about that patient.

No longer are medical records handwritten notes by the practitioner in the patient's file folder. Today medical records are electronic, enabling patient information to be available at anytime, anywhere depending on the availability of the electronic medical records system. Medical records are no longer kept on long shelves behind the reception desk in the practitioner's office or in oversized looseleaf binders in the chart room on the medical unit. Patients' records are stored in a database server (see Chapter 1) accessed by desktop and mobile computers over a computer network (see Chapter 7).

No longer can you feel and touch the patient's medical record. No longer is the patient's medical record in the exclusive custody of the practitioner.

Today the patient's medical record is stored at some remote location in a server that is overseen by nonclinicians. In some cases, the remote location is not owned by the healthcare facility.

This may seem disconcerting; however, the practice of storing sensitive information electronically in a remote location is commonplace in many industries because security controls can be uniformly imposed that provide at times greater security than is provided to the patient's medical records in a practitioner's office because there is a record of who accessed the information.

Electronic medical records are convenient to store and access and provide the opportunity to use state-of-the-art electronic protection of patient's records; however, there is also an increased risk for **unauthorized access**, identity theft, computer viruses, and denial of service attacks. Protection is provided by proxy servers, fire walls, encryption, and other means to secure the network, computing devices, and patient information.

1. Security Audit

A **security audit** is a process of reviewing a healthcare facility to identify security risks such as access to the facility. A component of the security audit is to review electronic and manual processes involved in recording, storing, and retrieving medical records. This includes **physical access** to the data center and computing devices along with electronic access to medical records.

There are two aspects to an informatics segment of the security audit. These are:

- Prevention of unauthorized access: Based on **Health Insurance Portability and Accountability Act (HIPAA)** regulations (see HIPAA and HITECH Act), only staff members who require access to patient information are authorized to access only the portion of the patient's information needed to perform their duties.
- **Information disclosure**: All staff members with authorized access to patient information must keep the information confidential. No staff member can share patient information with another unless that information is needed to perform their duties.

The informatics security audit must ensure the integrity of the information. Information must consistently be valid and processed correctly to deliver accurate information to the staff. The security audit must identify the risk if someone tampers with the information.

The informatics security audit begins with a review of policies and procedures that govern how patient information is maintained and accessed.

The audit should also identify electronic controls that facilitate access to the information and detect violations of policies and procedures. For example, security controls built into the application, database, or network verify that a login ID has access to patient information. Failed attempts to log in are electronically noted in a log and electronically reported to security officials for investigation.

Database Access Points

Auditors who perform the informatics security audit must identify **database access points**. A database access point is an entrance into the database that contains patient medical records. Patient medical records are stored electronically in a database located on a database server in the data center. The database is managed by database management system (DBMS), which is a software that stores and retrieves information. The DBMS is accessed by the electronic medical records application, which is used by the clinician to access the information.

There are three database access points here. The first is the database itself. A technician using certain software may be able to retrieve the patient's medical records directly from the database. The DBMS is the next access point. The DBMS responds to queries written in Structured Query Language (SQL) (see Chapter 4) that can be sent by any program or written interactively by a technician. The third access point is the electronic medical records application. The application sends SQL queries to the DBMS that accesses the information from the database. An additional database access point is the network. Clinicians connect to the database server over the network. An unauthorized person can also use the network to access the information.

A goal of an informatics security audit is to reduce the number of database access points. As a result, the threat to breach of the database is diminished.

Physical Access

Data servers, application servers, and other computing devices used to store and access patients' medical records should be housed in a secured location that is accessible by an authentication system. An authentication system is a system that controls access to secured facilities. Staff seeking access may require an electronically readable secured ID card or use biometrics such as a fingerprint reader to gain access to the facility.

An authentication system is not foolproof. For example, the authentication system will permit access to any electronically readable secured ID card that is encoded with the ID. This not does authenticate the person holding the card. Likewise, biometric readers typically have adjustable sensitivity controls that can be adjusted from 100% match to less than 50% match depending on the risk tolerance of the healthcare facility.

Password

ID and password combinations are the most commonly used authentication method to protect computer applications from unauthorized access. There is a continuing battle between intruders seeking to gain unauthorized access to a system and management information systems (MIS) department protecting access to the system. The challenge is to have staff create a password that is not easily guessed by intruders and yet be sure that the password is easy for the staff to remember.

Every system has a default password that should require the staff to change the password at the time of the initial login. However, administrator passwords to network software, operating systems, and other centrally managed application do not always require that the password be changed. Intruders know this and are able to log in as an administrator using the default password. Therefore, the security audit should determine if the default password was changed.

The MIS department typically sets policies for choosing a password. For example, common names are not permitted; the password must have uppercase and lowercase characters, must have a number, and must include a punctuation mark. You can imagine how frustrating it is for the staff to comply with the policy—and also how challenging it is to remember the password. Likewise, this is also challenging for intruders to guess the password, which is the point of the policy. Of course, there is a high likelihood that the staff will write down the password and place the password in a drawer or under the keyboard. Be sure to look in drawers and other common hiding places for passwords.

The MIS department should also require the staff to change the password frequently. In addition, the ID should be locked after a specific number of failed login attempts. The number of failed attempts will depend on the tolerance of the healthcare facility. Some facilities lock the ID after two attempts and require the employee to visit the security department to confirm the attempts before being permitted to reset the password. A failed attempt may indicate that the employee forgot the password or may indicate an attempt by an intruder to gain access to the system. Many healthcare facilities lock the ID after three or four attempts and permit the MIS department to have the employee reset the password based on a phone call to the helpdesk.

> **NURSING ALERT**
>
> The healthcare facility's password policy will depend on the probability that an intruder is likely to attempt to gain access using an employee's ID.

Disabling Services

A service is a feature of the operating system that enables an employee or a program to perform specific actions on the computing device. The MIS department should deactivate these features—called **disabling services**— because they can be used by intruders to gain unauthorized access to the computing device and related systems. Here are services that should be disabled:

- File transfer protocol (FTP) service: FTP is used to transfer files between computing devices over the Internet (see Chapter 7). FTP requires a login ID and password. The login ID can be any email address, and the password is anonymous. FTP should be disabled.

- File sharing: The operating system may have peer-to-peer services that enable two computing devices to share files. That is, a computing device will have access to local storage on the other computing device. File sharing services should be disabled.

2. HIPAA and HITECH Act

HIPAA was enacted in 1996 and imposed surety and privacy regulations for patients' medical records among other requirements. In 2009, the **Health Information Technology for Economic and Clinical Health (HITECH) Act** was passed that addressed privacy and security concerns related to the electronic transmission of patients' medical records.

HIPAA designated elements of patients' medical records that are considered protected health information, commonly referred to as **protected health identifiers (PHIs)**. PHIs can be accessed only for the purpose of caring for the patient. This is commonly referred to as the minimum necessary requirement. Furthermore, only the portion of PHIs needed to care for the patient can be accessed by those providing the care. For example, if a care provider does not need to know the patient's address to give care, then accessing the patient's address is a violation of HIPAA.

Table 10–1 lists 18 identifiers of personal health information that HIPAA designates as private and are protected under the HIPAA privacy rule.

TABLE 10–1 Eighteen HIPAA-Designated Protected Health Identifiers			
Names	Fax numbers	Health plan beneficiary number	Photos of the patient
Address	Email address	Account number	Any unique identifiers
Full zip code	Social security number	Vehicle identifiers	
All elements of data directly related to the patient	Medical record number	Universal resource locators (URLs)	
Telephone numbers	Visit number	Internet protocol (IP) address	

Sharing these identifiers with unauthorized personnel is a violation of HIPAA. Information can be shared if the patient signs a written consent authorizing that specific information can be shared with a specific person for a specific length of time. The consent formally is typically valid for 30 days.

NURSING ALERT

The first three digits of a zip code is not a PHI because the first three digits of the zip code usually identify an area of 20,000 people or more.

Permitted Disclosure

There are exceptions to disclosing PHIs that can be divided into four broad categories. These are:

- Patient treatment: PHIs and related healthcare information can be shared between providers for the purpose of treating the patient. The presumption is that the patient wants the information shared if the patient is unable to provide written consent.
- Payment for services: A healthcare provider can share PHIs with another healthcare provider to facilitate payment. That is, a practitioner can receive information about the practitioner's patient from a healthcare facility where the practitioner treated the patient.
- Healthcare operations: Administrators of a healthcare facility can use PHIs for training programs, personnel evaluations, and improving delivery of healthcare without the patient's written consent.

- Public welfare: PHIs can be shared with government agencies with a court order in public health emergencies. For example, a healthcare facility can share protected healthcare information with a government agency that is managing a bioterrorism emergency.

> **NURSING ALERT**
>
> Always confirm with the policies of the healthcare facility to know when PHIs can be shared with others.

The Omnibus Rule

The **Omnibus rule** for HIPAA increases patient privacy and security of the patient medical records. There are for major areas covered by the Omnibus rule. These are:

- **Business associates** covered: A business associate is any vendor used by the healthcare provider to manage patient medical records. A business associate is required to comply with HIPAA regulations. The business associate should conduct a security audit and certify to the healthcare provider that the business associate is HIPAA compliant.

- Sales of protected health information: Protected health information can be sold or used in marketing and fundraising purposes without authorization from the patient.

- Electronic copies of medical records: The patient has the right to receive an electronic copy of his or her medical records.

- Health plan restriction: The healthcare provider cannot disclose patient medical information to the patient's health plan for treatments paid for totally by the patient.

- Notification: A patient must be notified of a breach within 60 days of the breach of privacy.

Encryption and Destruction of Data

The HITECH Act requires that protected health information be encrypted (see Encryption) based on the class of information. The class of information describes the location of the data. There are four classes. These are:

- **Data at rest**: Data at rest is protected healthcare information stored on a server or other computing device. Several methods can be used to encrypt data at rest. These are:

- ° Full disk encryption: Full disk encryption requires that all data on the disk, including the operating system, be encrypted. Before installing the operating system in memory, which is called booting, the user is prompted to enter an ID and password. If authorized, the operating system is decrypted and loaded into memory.

- ° Virtual disk encryption: Virtual disk encryption groups files into a logical container. The content of the container is then encrypted. Only an authorized ID and password can gain access to the container and decrypt the contents of the container.

- ° Volume encryption: Volume encryption is the process of encrypting a section of the storage media called a volume. All files within the volume are encrypted. This is a commonly used encryption method for USB flash drives and hard drives.

- ° File or folder encryption: File or folder encryption is the process of encrypting the contents of a file or the contents of files that are logically organized into a folder on a storage device.

- **Data in motion**: Data in motion is protected healthcare information that is being transmitted over a network. Data can be encrypted at the network layer of the OSI model (see Chapter 7) using commercially available encryption software.

- **Data in use**: Data in use is protected healthcare information that is being created, retrieved, updated, or deleted. Privacy screens on monitors and restricted positioning of monitors away from public view are the best methods to protect data that is being used by staff.

- **Data disposed**: Data disposed is protected healthcare information that is being destroyed. The process of removing obsolete data is called sanitization. Deleting data from media does not remove the data. Data can be reconstructed. The sanitization process ensures that deleted data cannot be easily recovered. There are three commonly used methods for sanitizing data. These are:

- ° Clear: Clear is a method of overwriting the storage space with nonsensitive data using appropriate software and hardware.

- ° Purge: Purge is a method of degaussing. Degaussing is exposing the media to a strong magnetic field, causing disruption in the recorded data.

- ° Destroy: There are several methods for destroying the media. These are pulverization, melting, incineration, and shredding.

> ### NURSING ALERT
>
> If the media is not going to be reused, then the most cost-effective process is to destroy the media.

Compliant Checklist

Here are steps that can be taken to ensure that the healthcare facility is HIPAA compliant.

- Designate a staff member as the privacy security officer who is responsible to conduct security audits annually and ensure the facility policies and procedures are HIPAA compliant.
- Policies and procedures must be reviewed every 6 months to ensure HIPAA compliance.
- Train staff regularly on security and privacy compliance.
- Make sure all patient medical records are encrypted on all platforms, including mobile devices.
- Make sure all media is sanitized after data is obsolete.
- Make sure staff knows how to respond to breaches in security.

3. Proxy Servers

A healthcare facility network is commonly connected to the Internet, enabling the Internet to be accessed by computing devices within the healthcare facility. The connection between the Internet and the healthcare facility is facilitated by using a proxy server. A proxy server is an intermediary between the computing device within the healthcare facility that accesses the Internet website and the website itself. The computing device never directly interacts with the Internet.

The computing device uses a browser to connect to an Internet resource. The request for the Internet resource is sent over the healthcare facility's network to the proxy server. The proxy server notes the Internet Protocol (IP) address of the computing device and corresponding request. The proxy server then forwards the request to the website under the proxy server's IP address. All requests for Internet service sent by the healthcare facility use the proxy server's IP address. That is, the identity of the computing device that is accessing the website is hidden from the website.

> ### NURSING ALERT
>
> The proxy server can be configured to store the most frequently requested web pages in memory, called cache. Requests are then fulfilled from cache without having to send a request over the Internet. However, the cached web pages may not reflect the latest content on the web page.

Demilitarized Zone

The healthcare facility may provide information, such as clinic schedules, to those outside the healthcare facility. Information within the healthcare facility is kept within a secure area of the network with access protected in a number of ways (see HIPAA and HITECH Act and Firewall).

Information commonly shared with the community can be placed on a computing device or a segment of a computing device outside the security zone informally called the **demilitarized zone (DMZ)**. The segment of a computing device can be a directory on a disk drive. Computing devices outside the healthcare facility will access the healthcare facility over the Internet. Requests from the community are received by the proxy server. If the request is for unsecured information available in the DMZ, then the proxy server fulfills the request with information from the unsecured computing device.

4. Firewall

A firewall is a filter between the healthcare facility's network and computing devices connected to the network and the outside world such as the Internet. A firewall can be a computer program that filters all communication coming from the Internet and going to the Internet from computing devices on the network. A firewall might also be a detected computing device that filters communication based on rules established by the healthcare facility.

Information travels across the network in electronic envelops called packets (see Chapter 7). Packets destined for outside the healthcare facility's network pass through the firewall before reaching the proxy server. The firewall examines each packet and compares the content of the packet(s) with filtering rules. Based on the comparison, the packet is forwarded to the proxy server for processing or is rejected, causing an error message to be displayed on the browser of the computing device that generated the packet.

For example, the healthcare facility's committee on security and privacy may prohibit employees from accessing YouTube from computing devices within the healthcare facility. The MIS department sets the firewall to reject any packets destined for the YouTube IP address or the YouTube URL (see Chapter 7).

The firewall is also programmed to stop incoming messages from entering the healthcare facility's network by examining packets of each incoming message and comparing the packet(s) with the exclusion rules set by the MIS department. For example, certain IP addresses are from untrusted sources such as spammers. These can be blocked by the firewall before reaching the healthcare facility's network.

Firewall Controls Traffic Flow

There are three ways in which a firewall controls the flow of packets to ensure that the network and computing devices on the network are protected. These are:

- **Packet filtering**: Packet filtering is a method whereby the firewall compares the content of each packet with the filtering rules to determine if the packet should be passed along or rejected.

- **Stateful inspection**: Stateful inspection compares key elements of a packet—not the entire packet—with filtering rules to determine to reject or pass along the packet.

- Proxy server: A proxy server (see Proxy Server) can be incorporated into a firewall, enabling efficient filtering and transmission of packet.

> **NURSING ALERT**
>
> Filtering rules are typically stored in a database.

Configuring a Firewall

Filtering rules are used to configure a firewall to respond to incoming and outgoing transmissions. Filtering rules can allow or disallow the following transmissions:

- IP address: The firewall can block certain IP addresses or a range of IP addresses incoming and outgoing.

- Domain names: A domain name (see Chapter 7) is a name that corresponds to an IP address. Domain names can be blocked.

- Protocols: A protocol is a standard way of doing something such as transmitting packets. There are a variety of communication protocols (see Chapter 7). A firewall can be configured to block one or more protocols.

- Ports: A port is an entry point into a server. For example, port 80 is for web access, and port 21 is for FTP access. The firewall can block access to specific ports.

- Phrases: A list of words and phrases can be incorporated into the rules of a firewall, enabling the firewall to search through packets looking for matches. If there is a match, then the packet is rejected.

Breaking Through the Firewall

A firewall is a good line of defense; however, there are ways that some individuals try to circumvent the firewall protection. There are some common methods:

- Simple Mail Transfer Protocol (SMTP) session hijacking: SMTP is a common way email is transmitted over the Internet (see Chapter 7). An SMTP session is the active process of transmitting the email. Emails can be redirect by manipulating the SMTP server, making undesired email seem to be coming from a trusted source. That is, the email is received by the firewall with a trusted source's return address when in fact the email is coming from an untrusted source that is sent by spam or a virus (see Virus).

- Backdoors: A backdoor is a little known feature available in some applications that enables someone to circumvent security precautions. For example, a person is able run the application without having to enter an ID or password. Some programmers build backdoors into an application to facilitate development and testing.

- Source routing: Source routing occurs when a hacker makes packets appear to come from a trusted source by manipulating IP addresses within the packet.

- Remote login: A remote login enables a person to log into a computing device from another computing device. For example, the helpdesk technician uses a remote login to access a computer that is causing trouble for a user. After the user is remotely logged in, any data transmitted will appear to come from the local computer. Likewise, information received by the local computer can be seen and manipulated by the person who is remotely logged into the local computer.

5. Encryption

Encryption is the process of scrambling information called encoding so the information is not readable without decipher. A decipher is a device that unscrambles encrypted information called decoding. An encryption algorithm is used to define the way to scramble the information.

A key is a code used in a mathematical algorithm to encode and decode the information. Information is stored in a computing device in the form of bits (see Chapter 1). For example, "Jim" is stored as 01001010 01101001 01101101. A very simple key to encode information is to reverse each bit. That is, make 0 a 1 and 1 a 0. This is referred to as bit flipping. A computer application trying to read the encoded "Jim" will display strange characters on the screen, giving the impression that the file is corrupted. This is a very weak key.

56-bit key was used in the 1970s as the **Data Encryption Standard (DES)**. There can be 70 quadrillion combinations of 56 bits, making it nearly impossible to guess the key. However, speeds of computing devices have made this nearly impossible guess to reach the realm of probability.

The DES has been replaced by the **Advanced Encryption Standard (AES)**. The AES uses 128-bit key, 192-bit key, or 256-bit key, returning the ability to guess the key—even by a computer—to near impossible. Furthermore, Google is using a 2048-bit encryption key for the **Secure Socket Link (SSL)** certification system (see Digital Certificates).

Categories of Encryption

There are two categories of encryption. These are:

- **Symmetric key encryption**: A symmetric key encryption requires that the computing device receiving the encrypted information use the same key as the computing device that sends the encrypted information. A drawback of using symmetric key encryption is that computing devices receiving the encoded information must be known to the sender. This is problematic over the Internet when both computing devices are unknown to each other.

- **Asymmetric key encryption**: Asymmetric key encryption is commonly referred to as **public key** encryption and uses two keys to encode and decode information. These are the public key and the private key. Let's say that a remote computing device wants to send you encoded information. The remote computing device receives your computer's public key and uses the public key to encode the information. The encoded information is then transmitted to your computer. The private key on your computer is used to decode the information. The private key is known only to your computer. The public key cannot be used to decode the information.

NURSING ALERT

A popular encryption program is called Pretty Good Privacy (PGP) and can be used to encrypt any type of information.

Digital Certificates, SSL, and TLS

A digital certificate is a unique code issued by a known certificate authority certifying that a web server is trusted. That is, the web server is who it says it is. Each computer is provided with the public key of the other computer to transmit encrypted information.

Sensitive information is also transmitted over the Internet using SSL and **transport layer security (TLS)**. SSL is the original Internet security protocol that is replaced by the TLS. Both SSL and TLS use **digital certificates**.

When a request is made to transmit secure information, the http protocol changes to https, indicating that information will be transmitted securely. The browser initiating the transmission sends a digital certificate and the public key. The digital certificate is then verified for authenticity. The public key is then used to encode the information before sending the information to the browser.

A combination of asymmetric (public) key and symmetric key is used to facilitate secure transmission. The public key is used to send the symmetric key to the other computing device. The symmetric key is then used to encode information during the session. The symmetric key is then discarded at the end of the session. The symmetric key is only valid for the session.

Hash Value

A hash value is a value that is computed using a hashing algorithm and an input number. Hash values are used in public key encryption. Let's say that the input number that is to be encoded is 534. The hashing algorithm requires 534 to be multiplied by 143, producing the result of 76,362. 76,362 is then transmitted.

For a hacker to decode the 76,362, the hacker needs to know the multiplication factor (143). It is impossible to derive the multiplication factor from 76,362. However, the computing device receiving the transmission knows the multiplication value and can decode the transmission.

Public key encryption uses very large multiplication factors and more complex encryption algorithms, making it extremely unlikely that a computing device using brute force will be able to identify the hash value.

Authentication

Authentication is the process of verifying that a person has permission to access a computing device, data, or a facility. ID and password is the most common authentication method. A person is prompted to enter an ID and password, which are compared with the valid IDs and passwords. If there is a match, then the person is given access based on the security group assigned to the ID.

A security group is a logical grouping of IDs of people who have the same role within the healthcare facility. For example, practitioners assigned to a unit within the healthcare facility will have access to information about patients on that unit and have the right to write electronic orders for those patients using computerized physician order entry (CPOE). Registered nurses assigned to the same unit will belong to a different security group that give nurses access to patients' medical records but not access to CPOE. That is, nurses are not permitted to write electronic orders.

There are many security groups within a healthcare facility. The ID of a person can be assigned to many security groups depending on his or her role in the healthcare facility.

- Electronic ID cards is another commonly used authentication method. The ID card has a readable code. Each code is assigned to a security group. Based on the ID code, the card holder is granted or refused access to a facility.

- Biometrics is another method of authentication. A biometric reader scans a fingerprint, a retina, or the person's face. Some biometric devices are able to identify a person by the person's voice. Some employees believe that biometric recognition is too intrusive and are concerned that the biometric measurement can be used for purposes other than authentication.

- Digital signature is a widely accepted method of authenticating the person who originated an electronic document. The digital signature is a type of public key encryption that followed the digital signature standard (DSS) and uses the digital signature algorithm (DSA). After the electronic document is composed, the digital signature is applied to the document. The digital signature calculates a value based on the content of the document. The value remains with the document. Any changes to the electronic document after the digital signature is applied will change that value. The digital signature compares the value of the original electronic document with the value of the current document. The digital signature becomes invalid if these values are different, indicating that the document changed.

- The IP address from a sending computing device can be compared with a list of authorized IP addresses to ensure that the sending computer is authorized to access the receiving computing device. Transmission is rejected if the IP addresses are not validated.

> **NURSING ALERT**
>
> Authentication methods are not foolproof. An ID and password may be accurate, but the person entering them may not be authorized to do so. Electronic ID cards identify the card and not the holder of the card. Biometrics can be copied. Furthermore, the sensitivity of biometric readers can be adjusted. That is, fingerprint matches of 50% may be acceptable by the healthcare facility. IP addresses can be faked.

Cyclic Redundancy Check and Checksum

Cyclic redundancy check (CRC) and checksum are methods used to ensure that transmitted data is not corrupted during transmission. CRC and checksum are not used for encryption, although these methods can indicate if the data changed during transmission.

Checksum adds together bytes in a packet and places the sum in the packet trailer (see Chapter 7). The bytes in the packet are again added when the packet is received. The sum is compared with the sum in the trailer. If they match, then data has not changed. If they are different, the data has changed, and a request is made to resend the packet.

CRC uses a similar concept as checksum except polynomial division instead of addition is used to calculate bytes in the packet.

> **NURSING ALERT**
>
> For the best security, use technology that automatically generates session IDs and passwords and transmits packets encrypted with a secure shell (SSH) or using the AES.

6. Security on a Wireless Network

A wireless network (**Wi-Fi**) is used throughout healthcare facilities to extend the local area network without having to install cabling throughout the facility. Wi-Fi uses transceivers commonly called a hotspot placed in key locations that are connected to the network using cables. A transceiver sends and receives radio signals that are encoded with network packets (see Chapter 7). Any Wi-Fi–enabled computing device can receive and send information using the transceiver. Therefore, Wi-Fi transceivers must be secured.

Two common methods are used to secure a Wi-Fi connection. These are:

- Wi-Fi Protected Access Version 2 (WPA2): WPA2 uses either Temporal Key Integrity Protocol (TKIP) or AES to encode information transmitted over the Wi-Fi connection.
- Media access control (MAC): Every computing device capable of connecting to a network has a unique MAC address that is encoded into the computing device's network circuit (see Chapter 7). The Wi-Fi router can be configured to allow only specific MAC addresses to access the Wi-Fi connection. However, a hacker may be able to send a copy of the approved MAC address to the Wi-Fi to gain access. This is called spoofing.

> **NURSING ALERT**
>
> Be sure to disable the Wi-Fi Protected Setup (WPS) feature of the Wi-Fi router if possible. WPS makes setup easy; however, this feature is vulnerable to hackers.

Bluetooth Security

Bluetooth is a protocol that enables two devices to automatically establish a wireless connection using radio waves that are transmitted over a very short distance (see Chapter 7). Bluetooth is commonly used for hands-free connection between a headset and a cell phone. A Bluetooth connection has the same security risk as a Wi-Fi connection. That is, radio waves can be intercepted by another Bluetooth connection.

There are two ways to provide security on a Bluetooth device. These are:

- Nondiscoverable mode: A Bluetooth device can be placed in the nondiscoverable mode by the user, preventing other Bluetooth devices from connecting to the device. This is ideal if a user is not going to connect Bluetooth devices to the Bluetooth-enabled device.
- Trusted devices: A Bluetooth-enabled device can be configured to trust the source of data transmission. A trusted source can be given device level security, which is access to the device, or service level security (or both), which is access to specific data on the device. Most cell phones require authentication before giving access to a Bluetooth device.

7. Spam

Unsolicited commercial email, commonly referred to as spam, is unwanted messages sent to an email account. Spam is problematic for a healthcare facility because unless stopped, spam will reach every email account in the healthcare facility. Publicly available email providers such as AOL and Microsoft's Hotmail each block upwards of three billion spam per day. However, a healthcare facility usually does not use these services.

Spam is like an advertisement similar to junk mail. However, unlike junk mail, spam cost practically nothing to send. Companies that generate spam play the odds that a very small percentage of spam will be read and even a smaller percentage of those read will result in a sale. Although the percentage is small, the volume of spam sent is in the millions. Therefore, the number of actual sales is substantial, given the very low cost to send spam.

Although spam is an email, it is not sent the way you send an email. The spam email is formatted by a computer program using the email protocol (see Chapter 7). The computer program can generate thousands of emails per second.

Email Addresses

Email addresses are harvested by programs that search websites, chat rooms, and other sources where email addresses are publicly displayed. These programs are commonly referred to as spiders. A spider is a program that makes requests for web pages using the same protocol as is used by a browser. The web server sends the requested pages to the spider, thinking the spider is a browser. The web page consists of a markup language (hypertext markup language [HTML]) and text that is to appear on the screen. The markup langue tells the browser how to display the text.

The spider program searches each line of the web page looking for the @ symbol, which identifies text on either side of the @ symbol as an email address. The email address is then extracted and saved to a file later to be used by the program that generates the spam.

Email addresses are also purchased from organizations or retrieved from an organization's listing of employees or members. Spamming companies can assemble email addresses by manipulating names in the list to conform to the format of the organization's email address.

Preventing Spam

A firewall can be configured to disallow packets that contain suspected phrases. The trouble is that spammers tend to use less suspicious phrases in the subject line and in the text of the email. The healthcare facility can license software that filters spam. The software uses heuristic filters and Bayesian filters that apply a statistically based algorithm to determine if the email is spam.

Furthermore, providers of the software update the list of known spam phrases, increasing the likelihood that spam will be blocked.

There are organizations that provide lists of IP addresses that are used by companies that send spam. These IP addresses can be blocked, preventing packets coming from those IP addresses from entering the healthcare facility's network. However, spammers are quick to change IP addresses.

> **NURSING ALERT**
>
> The healthcare facility uses an Internet service provider (ISP) that provides a spam-blocking service at the ISP level before the spam reaches the healthcare facility.

8. Denial of Service Attack

Denial of service is a technique used by an unscrupulous person or group to prevent access to a computing device, typically a web server. Each computing device on a network has an IP address. On the healthcare facility's local area network, IP addresses are accessed by other computing devices on the network. The proxy server (see Proxy Server) is connected to both the local area network and with the Internet. The IP address of the proxy server is accessible by any computing device on the Internet.

A denial of service attack floods an IP address with packets so much so that packets sent by legitimate computing device are stuck in a traffic jam of packets. This is similar to a mailbox being stuffed with so much junk mail that the mail carrier is unable to deliver nonjunk mail to the address. The proxy server attempts to process each packet; however, the incoming volume of packets is beyond the capacity of the proxy server. Denial of service attacks can cause bottlenecks with the server that is under attack, connections to that server (increased bandwidth consumption), the firewall, the SQL server, and the load-balancing server.

Counter Attack

The proxy server forwards requests to the router (see Chapter 7) connected to the proxy server to process incoming requests. Routers are configured to discard packets from an IP address that floods the router with packets. The presumption is that the proxy server is under a denial of service attack by the computing device at that IP address. Knowing this defense, attackers send packets using various computing devices, each having its own IP address. Eventually, packets from these IP address will also be discarded.

Attackers are known to place programs in unsuspecting computing devices timed to execute a coordinated denial of service attack. There might be millions of computing devices, each with its own IP address, sending request to the proxy servicer's IP address. These programs are slipped onto unsuspecting computing devices as attachments to emails or part of download of files from the Internet.

NURSING ALERT

A defense to a denial of service attack is for the proxy server or computing device under attack is to send a TCP reply saying, "Window size equals 0." This tells the sending computer device that no new data can be received by the IP address. The denial of service attack may be suspended.

---

9. Identity Theft

Identity theft, commonly referred to as identity fraud, is the process of acquiring identification of another person and using the identification to impersonate that person. When a person's identification is stolen, the identification can be used for social program fraud, credit card fraud, and financial fraud, among other deceptive practices.

A healthcare facility is a prime source of personal information that may be exposed to identity theft. Patient information contains Social Security numbers and other personal identifiers that can be acquired and misappropriated by an identity thief.

Stolen Medical Benefits

A patient's medical benefits identifier is one of the most commonly misappropriated documents in healthcare facilities. The medical benefits identifier enables the identity thief to receive free medical benefits in the name of the other patient.

Fraudulent identification can be costly to the healthcare facility because the healthcare facility delivers services to the identity thief and then files reimbursement claims with the third-party payer. The third-party payer is likely to reject the claim if there is suspicion of identity theft.

Further complicating the situation is that patient records of the identity thief and the patient are comingled, resulting in misleading information. Test results for the identity thief are likely to be different from those of the patient. Treatments might be ordered based on inappropriate test results.

Reversing the Damage

Typically, the patient is the first to recognize that the patient's identity was stolen when the patient receives notices of services and charges that the patient did not incur. Sometimes a third party such as a credit card company notices unusual purchasing patterns and will notify the patient directly.

The patient faces an uphill challenge in reversing the consequences of the identity theft because the patient has to prove that he or she did not receive services and incur expenses associated with the service. Disputed claims are usually sent to collections rather than court, resulting in a negative impact on the patient's credit rating.

Protecting Against Identity Theft

The healthcare facility is the caretaker of patients' personal information and must devise systems that protect that information from staff and outsiders. The best approach is to store patient information electronically using encryption (see Encryption) and security groups to control access to the information.

All printed copies of electronic records should be placed in a burn box after use. A burn box is a locked box with a slit enabling papers to be dropped into the box. Papers can only be retrieved by unlocking the box. The contents of the box are removed and either burned or shredded.

Patient information that is in paper form must be kept in a secure place where access is strictly controlled and is under 24/7 watch by security cameras. No information should be permitted to be removed from the area without being inspected by security personnel.

Patients who require medical service or require access to their medical records must present two forms of state-issued photo identification in addition to the patient's medical benefits identification card. A copy of the photo identification should be retained in the patient's medical records. The patient's information and photo should be compared with the patient before service is rendered. The only exception is in emergencies. However, after the patient is out of crisis, the staff must verify the patient's identity.

10. Computer Viruses

Computer viruses are a major threat to the secure operations of electronic medical records because a computer virus might corrupt data or applications or maliciously disrupt the electronic medical records systems.

A computer virus is a small, malicious program that attaches to a file or application program. The computer virus activates when the file is opened or the application program runs whatever disruption that the computer virus programmer intended. The virus may also attach itself to other files and applications.

Trojan Horses and Worms

Two forms of computer viruses are called a **Trojan horse** and **worms**. A Trojan horse is a computer virus that appears to be a known file or application program. The unsuspecting user downloads the file or installs the application, causing the computer virus to activate. A Trojan horse does not replicate itself, although unsuspecting users might share the file or application program with others, enabling the Trojan horse to populate other computing devices.

A worm is a malicious program (computer virus) that exploits known weaknesses in network security, commonly referred to as a security hole. The worm searches for the security hole and then copies itself to networked computing devices and causes its intended disruption.

NURSING ALERT

A common way computer viruses are disrupted is as an attachment to email. When the email or the attachment is opened, the computer virus activates.

Inside a Computer Virus

A computer program is a set of instructions that is sent to the computer's central processor by the operating system for processing (see Chapter 1). A virus is a computer program that contains instructions telling the central processor to perform tasks that are unexpected and undesirable such as deleting files, changing the names of files, and copying files so that the storage media becomes full. A computer virus can do anything disruptive that can be imagined by the programmer who created the virus.

Think of a program as a series of instructions that are placed in a structured order on a disk. When the program runs, the operating system starts at the beginning of the program and loads instructions until the operating system reaches the end of the file. The programmer who writes a computer virus can write instructions to place the virus on the disk between the last instruction of the program and the end of the file. The operating system will then load the

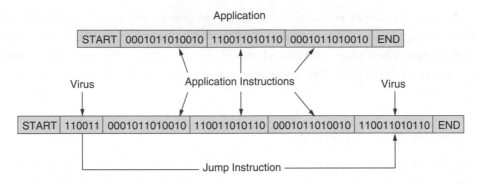

FIGURE 10-1 • A computer virus can be embedded into an application, causing the operating system to execute the computer virus when the application runs.

virus in memory as if the virus part of the instructions of the program. The operating system will eventually send instructions from the virus to the central processing unit as if those instructions were part of the program.

Some programmers who write computer viruses also replace one of the first instructions in the program with an instruction telling the operating system to jump to the viral portion of the program (Figure 10–1). This causes instructions of the computer virus to be processed ahead of the application's instructions.

Rootkit

A **rootkit** is a stealth program that is difficult to detect because the rootkit modifies programs designed to detect computer viruses. A rootkit is a computer virus that modifies administrative tools used to manage the operations of a computing device and causes the administrative tool to make inappropriate decisions.

A rootkit focuses on the operating system kernel. The kernel is the portion of the operating system that interacts with the computer hardware, boots the computer, loads programs and files, and directs the central processing unit.

NURSING ALERT

The kernel level of the operating system is the most trusted program running on a computing device. A rootkit corrupts the kernel, making the kernel untrustworthy. A rootkit is suspected based on unusual behavior of the computing device. Boot the computing device from a trusted copy of the operating system to determine if the suspected behavior changes. If so, then reinstall the operating system.

Computer Virus Protection

Virus detection software is the best way to protect against computer viruses entering a computing device. Makers of virus detection software identify the characteristics of known computer viruses. Characteristics include size, bit patterns, and how the computer virus infects a computing device.

New computer viruses are developed all the time. Makers of virus detection software actively investigate incidents of computer virus attacks and update the virus detection software immediately to limit attacks. The healthcare facility can receive nearly immediate updates depending on the licensing arrangement with the maker of the virus detection software.

Virus detection software scans all incoming files for known computer viruses before files are permitted on a computing device. The virus detection software automatically scans the computing device based on a schedule to assess if a computer virus has gained entrance to the computing device.

Computer viruses that are detected are isolated on the computing device. That is, the operating system will not access the computer virus. The virus detection software will then remove the computer virus.

> **NURSING ALERT**
>
> Virus detection software protects a computing device from known computer viruses based on a profile of computer viruses stored in the virus detection software. If the profile is not updated or if a computer virus is not known to the virus detection software, then the virus detection software will not protect the computing device from new computer viruses.

The MIS department must develop policies regarding who is authorized to download files and install applications on the healthcare facility's computing devices. Those policies must be enforced by controlling access to downloading and installing files and applications. Policies must strike a balance between protecting the healthcare facility's computing devices and enabling staff to conduct work efficiently. That is, staff will download files sent from outside the healthcare facility as part of the expected job function—and a computer virus may be attached to those files.

Macro Virus

A macro is a collection of interactions with an application—common in Microsoft Office—that is stored in a file under a file name commonly referred to as a macro name. The user runs the macro to execute those interactions.

This saves time when performing the same interactions frequently because you do not have to press all the keys. The macro does this for you.

A macro virus is a computer virus in the form of a macro. Executing the macro causes the application to execute interactions that may be destructive to the contents of application file (e.g., Word, Excel). Damage can be done before the user realizes that the macro virus is activated.

Make sure that the macro virus protection feature of the application is activated. This will reduce the likelihood of a macro virus attack.

NURSING ALERT

A computer virus can be attached as an executable files with the file extensions of EXE, COM, or VBS. Computer viruses can also be attached as JPG files.

CASE STUDY

CASE 1

As the nurse informatics specialist, you have been assigned to the team that will conduct the informatics security audit. The team is given the task of identifying weaknesses in the healthcare facility's informatics systems and processes and recommending ways that these can be strengthened. The informatics security audit must review all data in the healthcare facility, all applications, all computing devices, network devices, and policies and procedures that define how data, applications, and computing devices can be protected. The informatics security audit will assess electronic data and information stored on paper. The executive nurse asks the following questions about the informatics security audit. What are your best responses?

QUESTION 1. Where is a good starting point for the informatics security audit?
ANSWER: The team should begin by reviewing regulatory requirements set forth by regulatory authorities such as HIPAA and the HITECH Act and The Joint Commission. Regulatory authorities typically specify informatics security requirements and guidelines for conducting an informatics security audit. The team can use these guidelines as the foundation for the informatics security audit.

QUESTION 2. What patient information should be the focus of an informatics security audit?
ANSWER: The team should assess how all information is protected within the healthcare facility. However, particular attention needs to be given to how HIPAA-designated PHIs are protected by the healthcare facility. There are 18 PHIs (see Table 10–1).

QUESTION 3. What are the two main aspects of an informatics security audit?
ANSWER: These are prevention of unauthorized access to information, applications, and computing devices and information disclosure. Information disclosure is the process of how confidential information is released by the healthcare facility. Access and disclosure processes must be secured by placing controls in systems that authenticate the right of a staff member to access and share confidential information.

QUESTION 4. What should the team review in biometric devices used to authenticate staff?
ANSWER: The team should review the sensitivity settings of biometric devices. The sensitivity setting determines how the biometric device authenticates a staff member. The biometric device can be set at 100% match, requiring that the staff member's biometric exactly matches the corresponding biometric in the device's database. In reality, there is rarely a 100% match. Therefore, sensitivity is adjusted based on the healthcare facility's risk tolerance. That is, sensitivity can be adjusted to 50%, indicating that a staff member is authenticated with a 50% biometric match. The healthcare facility determines the appropriate tolerance. The team should simply report findings in the informatics security audit.

FINAL CHECK-UP

1. The executive nurse is reviewing a security audit performed by the MIS department. She asks you to explain the term *database access point*. What is the best answer?

   A. A database access point is an entrance into a computing device that displays patient medical records.

   B. A database access point is an entrance into a computing device that contains patient medical records.

   C. A database access point is an entrance into the database that contains patient medical records.

   D. A database access point is an entrance into application that contains a healthcare facility's records.

2. **The executive nurse asks you what is the goal of an informatics security audit. What is the best response?**

   A. A goal of an informatics security audit is to increase the number of database access points.

   B. A goal of an informatics security audit is to reduce the number of database access points.

   C. A goal of an informatics security audit is to identify the number of database access points.

   D. A goal of an informatics security audit is to identify who has access to a database access points.

3. **The director of MIS has been reading about protected health identifiers. She asks you to explain this term. What is the best response?**

   A. A personal health identifier is personal information about a patient that can never be shared with clinicians treating the patient without the patient's written or verbal consent under the HIPAA privacy rule.

   B. A personal health identifier is personal information about a patient that can never be shared with clinicians treating the patient without the patient's written consent under the HIPAA privacy rule.

   C. A personal health identifier is personal information about a patient that can be shared openly under the HIPAA privacy rule.

   D. A personal health identifier is personal information about a patient that is designated as private and is protected under the HIPAA privacy rule.

4. **The executive nurse is reading about the Omnibus rules and asks you to explain how these rules affect business associates. What is the best response?**

   A. A business associate is any vendor used by the healthcare provider to manage patient medical records.

   B. A business associate is any vendor used by the healthcare provider to manage patient medical records. A business associate is required to comply with HIPAA regulations.

   C. A business associate is any employee who manages patient medical records. A business associate is required to comply with HIPAA regulations.

   D. A business associate is any employee who manages patient medical records.

5. **The executive nurse is confused by the term *data in motion* in relation to protecting data. He asks you to explain this term. What is the best response?**

   A. Data in motion is protected healthcare information that is being transmitted over a network.

   B. Data in motion is protected healthcare information that is being stored on a network computing device.

   C. Data in motion is protected healthcare information that is being purged from a network computing device.

   D. Data in motion is protected healthcare information that is being cleared from a network computing device.

6. During a meeting, the executive nurse heard the director of MIS speak about a firewall. She asks you to explain this term after the meeting. What is the best response?

   A. A firewall is a router that connects the healthcare facility's network to the Internet.

   B. A firewall is a computing device that routes information over the network.

   C. A firewall is a computing device that connects to the network and the outside world such as the Internet.

   D. A firewall is a filter between the healthcare facility's network and computing devices connected to the network and the outside world such as the Internet.

7. The executive nurse reads that a key is used to encode information that is stored or transmitted over a network. He asks you to explain the concept of a key. What is the best response?

   A. A key is used to unlock the encryption algorithm used to encode and decode the information.

   B. A key is a code used in a mathematical algorithm to encode and decode the information.

   C. A key is a term used to describe encrypted information.

   D. A key is used to protect encrypted information that is sent over the network.

8. The executive nurse is reading an article about digital certificates and asks you to explain this concept. What is the best response?

   A. A digital certificate is a unique code issued by the MIS department that certifies that a web server is trusted.

   B. A digital certificate is a unique code issued by the healthcare facility that certifies that a web server is trusted.

   C. A digital certificate is a unique code issued by a known certificate authority certifying that a web server is trusted.

   D. A digital certificate is a unique code issued by the Internet standards body that certifies that a web server is trusted.

9. The executive nurse heard on the news that a government website was the target of a denial of service attack. She asks you to explain denial of service attack. What is the best response?

   A. Denial of service prevents the MIS department access to the healthcare facility's web server.

   B. Denial of service is a technique used to prevent access to a web server by sending very large numbers of requests to the web server, preventing others from accessing the web server.

   C. Denial of service prevents some patient access to the healthcare facility's web server.

   D. Denial of service prevents some staff member access to the healthcare facility's web server.

10. **The executive nurse asks you what the primary risk is for identity theft for the healthcare facility. What is the best response?**

   A. Theft of a patient's visit number

   B. Theft of patient credit card information

   C. A patient presenting another patient's medical benefits information when requesting medical care by the healthcare facility

   D. Thefts of a patient's medical records number

CORRECT ANSWERS AND RATIONALES

1. C. A database access point is an entrance into the database that contains patient medical records.
2. B. A goal of an informatics security audit is to reduce the number of database access points.
3. D. A personal health identifier is personal information about a patient that is designated as private and is protected under the HIPAA privacy rule.
4. B. A business associate is any vendor used by the healthcare provider to manage patient medical records. A business associate is required to comply with HIPAA regulations.
5. A. Data in motion is protected healthcare information that is being transmitted over a network.
6. D. A firewall is a filter between the healthcare facility's network and computing devices connected to the network and the outside world such as the Internet.
7. B. A key is a code used in a mathematical algorithm to encode and decode the information.
8. C. A digital certificate is a unique code issued by a known certificate authority certifying that a web server is trusted.
9. B. Denial of service is a technique used to prevent access to a web server by sending very large numbers of requests to the web server, preventing others from accessing the web server.
10. C. A patient presenting another patient's medical benefits information when requesting medical care by the healthcare facility.

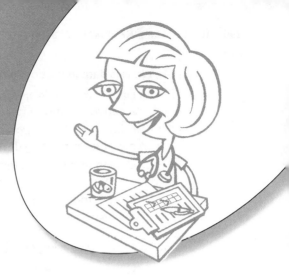

Final Exam

1. **Why would you use a TRANSACTION statement?**
   A. A TRANSACTION statement defines a transaction application.
   B. A TRANSACTION statement defines a group of SQL statements that form a transaction.
   C. A TRANSACTION statement creates a transaction database.
   D. A TRANSACTION statement creates a transaction table.

2. **A colleague who is taking a nursing informatics course asks you to explain how digital information is encoded on an analog wave. What is the best response?**
   A. The wave's length determines the binary value.
   B. The wave's frequency determines the binary value.
   C. The wave's peak is considered a binary 1, and a wave's trough is considered a binary 0.
   D. An analog wave cannot be encoded with digital data.

3. **What is a good faith negotiation?**
   A. Negotiating in good faith means that a party is at the breakpoint.
   B. Negotiating in good faith means that a party is not sincerely interested in reaching an agreement.
   C. Negotiating in good faith means that a party is sincerely interested in reaching an agreement.
   D. Negotiating in good faith means that the vendor is at the breakpoint.

4. **What is data in motion in relation to protecting data?**

   A. Data in motion is protected healthcare information that is being cleared from a network computing device.

   B. Data in motion is protected healthcare information that is being stored on a network computing device.

   C. Data in motion is protected healthcare information that is being purged from a network computing device.

   D. Data in motion is protected healthcare information that is being transmitted over a network.

5. **You colleague asks you where queries are written. What is the best response?**

   A. Queries are entered into an SQL console.

   B. Queries are embedded into programs or entered into an SQL console.

   C. Queries are embedded into programs.

   D. Queries are written by the clinical staff to retrieve information from the database.

6. **The MIS director said that the CPOE must use real-time processing. A nurse manager who attended the meeting asks you what the MIS director means by that term. What is the best response?**

   A. All processing is processed at the same time, and results are immediate.

   B. All processing is processed at the same time, and results are delayed.

   C. Information is processed as the information is received. The processing result is immediate.

   D. Information is processed as the information is received. The processing result is delayed.

7. **How can you summarize data in a query?**

   A. Use the VALUES clause

   B. Use the WHERE clause

   C. Use the FROM clause

   D. Use Column Functions

8. **A colleague asks you to explain how timing can be a barrier to effective communication. What is the best response?**

   A. The person receiving the message will always have sufficient time to understand the message.

   B. The person sending the message may not have sufficient time to convey the message.

   C. The person sending the message may not have time to tell the receiver what the receiver is expected to do with the information.

   D. The person receiving the message may not be in the frame of mind to listen and understand the message.

9. **What is a legacy system?**

   A. A legacy system is a process that has not been reviewed or upgraded for a long time but provides an important process in the operations of the healthcare facility.

   B. A legacy system is a system provided by a vendor.

   C. A legacy system is an older version of the current system that is important to the operations of healthcare facility.

   D. A legacy system is the new version of a system that is important to the operations of the healthcare facility.

10. **Who is in charge during a disaster?**

    A. Each unit manager

    B. The president of the healthcare facility

    C. The chief operating office of the healthcare facility

    D. The emergency incident commander

11. **The executive nurse asks you what is cost of ownership. What is the best response?**

    A. Cost of ownership is the total cost of acquiring and using a good or service.

    B. Cost of ownership is the total cost of using a good or service.

    C. Cost of ownership is the purchase price of an electronic medical records system.

    D. Cost of ownership is the total cost of acquiring a good or service.

12. **Why would you celebrate the failure of a member of the project team?**

    A. Celebration acknowledges that the team member attempted to do the correct thing.

    B. Celebration encourages the team member to try harder next time.

    C. Knowing what does not work is just as important as knowing what does work.

    D. Celebration helps to maintain self-esteem.

13. **The executive nurse asks you when the user acceptance test should be developed. What is the best response?**

    A. At the half-way point in the project

    B. Near the end of the project

    C. At the start of the project

    D. Before the project begins

14. **How do you remove duplicate values in a query?**

    A. Distinct clause

    B. Column functions

    C. GROUP BY clause

    D. HAVING clause

15. **What metric would you use to measure efficiency of data capture?**

    A. The number of clicks to perform a task to the minimum.
    B. Let stakeholders design the system.
    C. Let a clinical systems designer design data capture without input from stakeholders.
    D. Let a clinical systems designer design data capture with input from stakeholders.

16. **The nurse uses the term *system* to speak only about a computer application. You point out that a system is more than a computer application. What is the best description of a system?**

    A. A system is computer hardware.
    B. A system is a way of using a computer to do something to achieve a desired result.
    C. A system is a way of doing something to achieve a desired result.
    D. A system is computer hardware and software.

17. **Describe when you would use Agile project methodology.**

    A. Agile project methodology is used for relatively small, complex projects that can be accomplished by a team of up to nine members who are cross-functional.
    B. Agile project methodology is used for projects that require flexibility.
    C. Agile project methodology is used for relatively large, complex projects that can be accomplished by a team of up to nine members who are cross-functional.
    D. Agile project methodology is used for relatively small, routine, less complex projects that can be accomplished by a team of up to nine members who are cross-functional.

18. **What is the IP address 255.255.255.255?**

    A. APIPA
    B. Loopback address
    C. Default network
    D. Network broadcast

19. **What is a goal of the informatics security audit?**

    A. A goal of an informatics security audit is to increase the number of database access points.
    B. A goal of an informatics security audit is to reduce the number of database access points.
    C. A goal of an informatics security audit is to identify the number of database access points.
    D. A goal of an informatics security audit is to identify who has access to a database access point.

20. **What is the difference between a natural disaster and a human-made disaster?**

    A. A natural disaster is caused by an accident. A human-made disaster is caused by an unintentional or intentional act of a person.

    B. A natural disaster is caused by an act of nature. A human-made disaster is caused by not preparing for the natural disaster.

    C. A natural disaster is caused by an act of nature. A human-made disaster is caused by an unintentional or intentional act of a person.

    D. A natural disaster is caused by preventable act of nature. A human-made disaster is caused by an unintentional or intentional act of a person.

21. **During an interview for a nurse informatics analyst position, the interviewer asks you to explain the term *packet switching*. What is the best response?**

    A. The transfer of packets inside a computing device

    B. OSI model

    C. The transfer of packets between networks

    D. A circuit in a fiber optic network

22. **The executive nurse asks you to explain the term *mediation*. What is the best response?**

    A. Mediation is a process during which the mediator decides the disputed issue.

    B. Mediation is the process of avoiding conflicts.

    C. Mediation is a process during which the mediator helps two sides find common ground.

    D. Mediation is the process of making decisions.

23. **A colleague who is taking a nursing informatics course asks you what duration is. What is the best response?**

    A. Duration is the time required to begin the project.

    B. Duration is the length of the project.

    C. Duration is the time necessary to create the project charter.

    D. Duration is the length of time resources work on a task plus elapsed time.

24. **A nurse manager who recently joined the steering committee read an MIS report about data modeling. He asks you to explain this term. What is the best response?**

    A. Data modeling is a method used to design the data output for a clinical database application.

    B. Data modeling is a method used to design the data input for a clinical database application.

    C. Data modeling is a method used to define data requirements of a clinical process and identify relationship between data elements.

    D. Data modeling is a method used to design the data output and input for a clinical database application.

25. **A new nurse who is interested in nursing informatics asks you to explain the concept of word breakdown structure. What is the best response?**

    A. Dividing tasks among resources.

    B. A process of creating a complex system from small components.

    C. A process of decomposing a simple request into smaller and smaller components that are easy to comprehend and analyze.

    D. Breaking down tasks into milestones.

26. **A new nurse heard that the healthcare facility is going to get government funds to improve technology related to patient care. He asks you what the program is called. What is the best response?**

    A. Electronic medical records

    B. HITECH Act

    C. Meaningful use

    D. CPOE

27. **A colleague is taking a course in nursing informatics and asks you to explain SQL. What is the best response?**

    A. SQL is a DBMS that stores and manipulates clinical data.

    B. SQL is a type of database specifically designed to retrieve and manipulate clinical information.

    C. SQL is a type of programming language designed to build database applications.

    D. SQL is a type of programming language specifically designed to interact with DBMS to retrieve and manipulate information in the clinical database.

28. **Why is it important for you know group dynamics?**

    A. Group dynamics is used by the nurse informatics project manager to interact with patients.

    B. Group dynamics principles assist the nurse informatics project manager address the needs of the project sponsor.

    C. Group dynamics is a management tool that helps the nurse informatics project manager assign tasks to resources.

    D. Understanding of group dynamics can help the nurse informatics project manager keep the project team and stakeholders focused on the project.

29. **Explain the term *arbitrator*.**

    A. An arbitrator meets with both parties to identify all facts related to negotiations.

    B. An arbitrator meets with both parties to identify facts that are in dispute.

    C. An arbitrator unilaterally settles disputes.

    D. An arbitrator helps both parties settle a dispute.

30. What is a denial of service attack?

A. Denial of service prevents the MIS department from accessing the healthcare facility's web server.

B. Denial of service is a technique used to prevent access to a web server by sending very large numbers of requests to the web server, preventing others from accessing the web server.

C. Denial of service prevents some patients access to the healthcare facility's web server.

D. Denial of service prevents some staff members access to the healthcare facility's web server.

31. What is the difference between a disaster recovery plan and business continuity plan?

A. A disaster recovery plan focuses on restoring operations. Healthcare facilities do not have business continuity plans because a healthcare facility is not a business.

B. A disaster recovery plan focuses on restoring clinical operations. A business continuity plan focuses on restoring business operations.

C. A disaster recovery plan focuses on restoring both clinical and business operations. A business continuity plan is not needed for a healthcare facility.

D. A disaster recovery plan focuses on restoring operation during the first week of the disaster. A business continuity plan focuses on restoring operations after the first week of the disaster.

32. What code is used to encode characters so that the characters can be transmitted over the network?

A. Binary

B. ASCII

C. Decimal

D. Hex

33. What is a sprint in an Agile project?

A. A sprint is an activity performed by an Agile project team to groom the backlog of stories on the focus board.

B. A sprint is an activity performed by an Agile project team to set priorities of stories.

C. A sprint is a unit of work that lasts a fixed duration such as 1 week but can be upwards to 1 month.

D. A sprint is a unit of work that lasts a variable duration such as 1 week but can be upwards to 1 month.

34. **How is search criteria specified in a query?**
    A. Use the FROM clause
    B. Use the SELECT clause
    C. Use the WHERE clause
    D. Use the VALUES clause

35. **During an interview for a nurse informatics position, the interviewer asks you to explain the purpose of a foreign key. What is the best response?**
    A. A foreign key is a primary key of another table and is used to define an independent clinical relationship among data.
    B. A foreign key is a primary key of another table and is used to define a dependent relation.
    C. A foreign key is a foreign key of another table and is used to define a dependent relation.
    D. A foreign key is a primary key of another table and is used to define an independent relationship among data.

36. **A nurse manager watches you creating a leveling diagram and wonders what you are doing. What is the best response?**
    A. To better understand the workflow.
    B. To describe the work breakdown structure.
    C. To discuss elements of the system with different clinicians.
    D. A leveling diagram is a data flow diagram that gradually breaks down a process into details of the process.

37. **The nurse manager became confused when the MIS director spoke of an electronic medical administration records system as a transaction processing system. The nurse manager believes a transaction processing system involves purchasing goods. What is a good response?**
    A. A transaction processing system assists the manager in making decisions by analyzing information stored in a database.
    B. A transaction processing system is designed to provide information to assist the manager in making decisions.
    C. A transaction processing system is a system that stores and retrieves data and is usually integrated with other types of systems.
    D. A transaction processing system captures, processes, and stores information.

38. **A new nurse is taking an informatics course and asks you to explain the term *DBMS*. What is your best response?**
    A. A database management system is a computer application that manages access to clinical information stored in several database applications.
    B. A database management system is a computer application that manages information stored in the database

C. A database management system is a computer application that gives patients access to their clinical information admissions information from home.

D. A database merger system is a computer application that merges information stored in several database applications.

39. **A colleague is looking at a list of tasks and wonders what a task is. What is the best response?**

    A. A task is something someone does.

    B. A task is an element of a milestone.

    C. A task is an element of the project charter.

    D. A task is an action that has a beginning and an end that produces a result.

40. **How would you explain the term *CSMA/CD*?**

    A. To detect network traffic and collisions of nodes

    B. To detect network traffic and collision of MAC on the network

    C. To detect network traffic

    D. To detect network traffic and collisions of packets

41. **The executive officer asks you to explain the meaning of value as related to negotiations. What is the best response?**

    A. Value is expected performance when the contract is executed.

    B. Value is the promise the vendor makes to the healthcare facility to deliver a product or service.

    C. Value is the perception of worth. The perception of value is used in negotiation to create a relatively low-cost incentive to reach the terms of a contract.

    D. Value is time spent negotiating with the vendor.

42. **What is risk tolerance regarding risks associated with a disaster?**

    A. Risk tolerance is the amount of risk that the administrator is comfortable with accepting related to a risk associated with a disaster.

    B. Risk tolerance is a response to risk.

    C. Risk tolerance is a measurement of how often a computing device will fail.

    D. Risk tolerance is a measurement of how long a computing device will operate before the computing device fails.

43. **What is a digital certificate?**

    A. A digital certificate is a unique code issued by the MIS department that certifies that a web server is trusted.

    B. A digital certificate is a unique code issued by the healthcare facility that certifies that a web server is trusted.

    C. A digital certificate is a unique code issued by a known certificate authority certifying that a web server is trusted.

    D. A digital certificate is a unique code issued by the Internet standards body that certifies that a web server is trusted.

44. **What is a progress payment?**

    A. A progress payment is a payment for future work that the vendor will perform during the project.

    B. A progress payment is payment for capital expenses incurred by the vendor during the project.

    C. A progress payment is payment for noncapital expenses incurred by the vendor during the project.

    D. A progress payment is payment to the vendor for work completed during the project.

45. **How many network segments are connected by a router?**

    A. Two

    B. 256

    C. 255

    D. An endless number of segments

46. **The executive nurse asks you the purpose of the RACI chart. What is the best response?**

    A. The RACI chart identifies tasks that have a direct impact on the project deadline.

    B. The RACI chart describes when tasks are scheduled to be performed.

    C. The RACI chart identifies responsibility and accountability and who has to be consulted and informed about the project.

    D. The RACI chart identifies the organization chart of the project.

47. **Your colleague who is taking a nursing informatics course asks you to explain a stored procedure. What is the best response?**

    A. A stored procedure is a frequently used query that is stored within a clinical database application.

    B. A stored procedure is a query that resides on the DBMS.

    C. A stored procedure is a frequently used query.

    D. A stored procedure is a query that resides on the DBMS and can be executed by calling the name of the stored procedure in an SQL statement.

48. **The MIS director used to phrase instance of an entity. The executive nurse was confused and asks you to explain. What is the best response?**

    A. An instance of an entity is data associated with the entity.

    B. An instance of an entity consists of rows and columns.

    C. An instance of an entity is a collection of patient information.

    D. An instance of an entity consists of columns.

49. **What role arranges funding for the clinical system and determines what the system will do?**

    A. Programmer
    B. Project manager
    C. Stakeholder
    D. System owner

50. **The MIS director tells the executive nurse that the CPOE system will be placed on an application server. The executive nurse asks you to explain the term *application server*. What is the best response?**

    A. It is a computer that enables multiple users to save and use files to the same disk.
    B. It is a computer that runs a database management system (DBMS).
    C. It is a computer that manages the computer network.
    D. It is a computer where applications are stored and distributed from when requested by users.

51. **The MIS manager of computer hardware briefed the steering committee on the database server. The executive nurse is on the steering committee and does not understand the term *database server* and asks you to explain. What is the best response?**

    A. A database server is a DBMS used to store patient information.
    B. A database server is a network connection that enables computers outside the healthcare facility to access the database.
    C. A database server is a network connection that enables computers throughout the healthcare facility to access the database.
    D. A database server is a computer connected to a network that enables computers throughout the healthcare facility to access the database.

52. **The executive nurse heard the MIS director speak about a project charter and asks you to explain that term. What is the best response?**

    A. A project charter specifies responsibilities for stakeholders.
    B. A project charter specifies what the project manager is to deliver and the terms under which the project manager will manage the project.
    C. A project charter specifies all tasks associated with the project.
    D. A project charter specifies what the project manager is to deliver and the terms under which the project manager will manage the project.

53. **What is the purpose of a virtual team?**

    A. A virtual team is a project team that communicates using video conferencing and email.
    B. A virtual team is a project team on which the participants remain for the length of the project.
    C. A virtual team is a project team in which the participants join to complete a specific task and then leave the team after the task is completed.
    D. A virtual project team is a group of participants who move as a unit through a series of projects.

54. **What are the common failures of procurement?**

    A. Clearly define specifications
    B. Detail specifications
    C. Poor planning in negotiations
    D. Over- or understatement of work

55. **What is a data synchronization point?**

    A. The data synchronization point is when data is used by the MIS department.
    B. The data synchronization point is when data is used by end users.
    C. The data synchronization point is when data is restored.
    D. The data synchronization point is when data is backed up.

56. **How is a key used to encode information that is stored or transmitted over a network?**

    A. A key is used to unlock the encryption algorithm used to encode and decode the information.
    B. A key is a code used in a mathematical algorithm to encode and decode the information.
    C. A key is a term used to describe encrypted information.
    D. A key is used to protect encrypted information that is sent over the network.

57. **What options are available to respond to a risk?**

    A. Accept, mitigate, transfer, and avoid
    B. Accept, mitigate, and avoid
    C. Accept, transfer, and avoid
    D. Accept, mitigate, transfer, submit, and avoid

58. **Your colleague who is taking a nursing informatics course asks you to explain the term *node*. What is the best response?**

    A. A device connected directly to a switch
    B. A device connected directly to a router
    C. A device connected to the network
    D. A device connected directly to bridge

59. **Why would you use SBAR?**

    A. SBAR is a framework for mobile communications with practitioners.

    B. SBAR is a framework for describing a critical situation.

    C. SBAR is used for practitioners to communicate with other practitioners.

    D. SBAR is a framework for communicating effectively so decisions can be made quickly.

60. **How would you combine tables in a query?**

    A. Using a dataflow diagram

    B. Using a join

    C. Using naming conventions

    D. Using the ORDER BY statement

61. **What is an important concept in a relational database design?**

    A. In a relational database design, most duplicate information is removed from the database.

    B. In a relational database design, all conflicts with clinical information are resolved before the information is stored in the database.

    C. In a relational database design, clinical information can be stored in multiple databases.

    D. In a relational database design, only authorized staff members are able to access clinical information.

62. **The executive heard the MIS director speak about stakeholders. She asks, "What is a stakeholder?" What is the best response?**

    A. A stakeholder is any clinician who has an interest in an existing or proposed clinical information system.

    B. A stakeholder is any person who has an interest in an existing or proposed clinical information system.

    C. A stakeholder is any patient who has an interest in an existing or proposed clinical information system.

    D. A stakeholder is any administrator who has an interest in an existing or proposed clinical information system.

63. **A new registered nurse is interested in becoming a nurse informatics specialist. She asks you to describe the role of the nurse informatics specialist. What is your best response?**

    A. Consultant, educators researcher, and analyst

    B. Programmer, analyst, MIS coordinator, and nurse

    C. Policy developer, analyst, nurse supervisor, and programmer

    D. Consultant, analyst, and nurse coordinator

64. **The executive nurse read in an MIS report about using a clinical database. She asks you to explain the term. What is your best response?**

   A. A clinical database is a database server used to store clinical information.

   B. A clinical database is a computer program that is used to store and retrieve patient information or information necessary for patient care.

   C. A clinical database is a computer application that is used to store and retrieve patient information or information necessary for patient care.

   D. A clinical database is the electronic repository of patient information or information necessary for patient care.

65. **Why would you use stored procedures?**

   A. Stored procedures are required by HIPAA to protect access to patient information.

   B. A stored procedure is a requirement of all clinical information systems.

   C. A stored procedure reduces the transmission time necessary to execute a query.

   D. A stored procedure is a way a clinical application complies with HIPAA.

66. **How would you use the stages of adoption?**

   A. The stages of adoption is the process of developing the project charter.

   B. The stages of adoption is the process of hiring a member of the project team.

   C. The stages of adoption is a process for adopting a proposal.

   D. The stages of adoption is the process the project sponsor uses to accept the product of the project.

67. **The executive nurse asks you to explain the term *computing device*. What is the best response?**

   A. It is any device on a wireless network.

   B. It is any device that can calculate.

   C. It is any device that can interact with a network.

   D. It is any device that connects to Wi-Fi.

68. **The executive nurse is confused when you mentioned the term *method* of an object. What is the best way to clarify this term?**

   A. A method is used to define an object.

   B. A method is used to define an entity.

   C. A method is used to define an attribute.

   D. A method is a behavior of an object.

69. **Which of the following is the best description of a clinical information system?**

    A. A clinical information system is data that is processed, stored, and needed to care for a patient.
    B. A clinical information system is an arrangement of patients and the patients' medical teams, data, processes, and information technology that interacts to collect, process, store, and provide as output the information needed to care for the patients.
    C. A clinical information system is patient information stored in a database.
    D. A clinical information system is an electronic medical record system.

70. **During the steering committee meeting, an MIS analyst was discussing the concept of referential integrity. The executive nurse asked you to explain this concept. What is the best response?**

    A. Referential integrity occurs when a foreign key value is similar to a primary key value in a relation.
    B. Referential integrity occurs when a foreign key value matches a primary key value in a relation.
    C. Referential integrity occurs when a foreign key value does not match a primary key value in a relation.
    D. Referential integrity occurs when a foreign key value is substantially different than a primary key value in a relation.

71. **Your colleague wonders why is it important to use a naming convention. What is the best response?**

    A. A naming convention standardizes how names of columns are written, making the names easy for the person writing or reading the query to read and identify the kind of information stored in the column.
    B. Naming conventions are required by the DBMS.
    C. A naming convention standardizes how names of columns are written, making the names easy to read and making it easy to identify the kind of information stored in the column.
    D. A naming convention standardizes how names of columns are written, making the names easy for the DBMS to read and making it easy to identify the kind of information stored in the column.

72. **Why would you form a steering committee?**

    A. The steering committee is a group of nurses who provide input to the project.
    B. The steering committee is a group of clinicians who are responsible for the project.
    C. The steering committee is a group of influential leaders who act as a sounding board for the nurse informatics specialist during the life of the project.
    D. The steering committee is a group of clinicians who oversee development of the project.

73. **Which of the following is an example of a disincentive?**

    A. The healthcare facility will penalize the vendor 1% of the price for each month over the scheduled deadline.

    B. The healthcare facility will give the vendor 1% of the price for each month the system is delivered before the scheduled deadline.

    C. The healthcare facility will give the vendor 1% of the price for delivering the system on schedule.

    D. The healthcare facility will walk away from the contract.

74. **What is a firewall?**

    A. A firewall is a router that connects the healthcare facility's network to the Internet.

    B. A firewall is a computing device that routes information over the network.

    C. A firewall is a computing device that connects to the network and the outside world such as the Internet.

    D. A firewall is a filter between the healthcare facility's network and computing devices connected to the network and the outside world such as the Internet.

75. **What is a service level of agreement?**

    A. A service level of agreement is a contract that specifies the maximum level of service that a vendor will provide to the healthcare facility.

    B. A service level of agreement is an understanding that specifies the minimal level of service that a vendor will provide to the healthcare facility.

    C. A service level of agreement is a contract that specifies the minimal level of service that a vendor will provide to the healthcare facility.

    D. A service level of agreement is an understanding that specifies the maximum level of service that a vendor will provide to the healthcare facility.

76. **The MIS director asks you to explain the primary benefit of IMAP. What is the best response?**

    A. Emails remains on the email server.

    B. Emails cannot be deleted.

    C. Emails remain in cache.

    D. Emails remain on the local computer.

77. **The MIS analyst was explaining the physical database design during a steering committee meeting. The executive nurse asks you to explain this concept. What is the best response?**

    A. A physical database design contains technical specifications for linking tables.

    B. A physical database design contains technical specifications for linking data.

    C. A physical database design contains technical specifications for storing data.

    D. A physical database design contains technical specifications for storing indexes.

78. **The executive nurse heard the MIS director speak of a systems integrator. She asks you to explain this term. What is your best response?**

    A. It identifies new technological solutions to clinical problems.
    B. It incorporates technology in the facilities policies and procedures.
    C. It assesses technology needed for the clinic.
    D. It ensures that all clinical systems are able to work together.

79. **What is a personal health identifier?**

    A. A personal health identifier is personal information about a patient that can never be shared with clinicians treating the patient without the patient's written or verbal consent under the HIPAA privacy rule.
    B. A personal health identifier is personal information about a patient that can never be shared with clinicians treating the patient without the patient's written consent under the HIPAA privacy rule.
    C. A personal health identifier is personal information about a patient that can be shared openly under the HIPAA privacy rule.
    D. A personal health identifier is personal information about a patient that is designated as private and is protected under the HIPAA privacy rule.

80. **What are detective measures in the disaster recovery plan?**

    A. Detective measures are processes that focus on the occurrence of the disaster.
    B. Detective measures are processes that discovered that a disaster occurred.
    C. Detective measures are processes that restore function to the healthcare facility during or after a disaster.
    D. Detective measures are processes that prevent a disaster from occurring.

81. **The executive nurse asks you to explain the term *network packet*. What is the best response?**

    A. Fiberoptic transmission
    B. Email
    C. An electronic envelop used to transmit frames over the network
    D. An electronic envelop used to transmit information over the network

82. **Why would you use a risk management plan?**

    A. The risk management plan identifies risks associated with project development and defines how the nurse informatics project manager will address each risk.
    B. The risk management plan identifies risks associated with the clinical application and defines how each risk will be addressed.
    C. The risk management plan identifies risks associated with the healthcare facility and defines how each risk will be addressed.
    D. The risk management plan identifies risks associated with the healthcare industry and defines how each risk will be addressed.

83. **The executive nurse returned from a meeting with the MIS director where the term *milestone* was discussed. She asks you what a milestone is. What is the best response?**

    A. A milestone is a reportable finding to stakeholders by the project manager.

    B. A milestone is a measurement of significant progress.

    C. A milestone is an output of an action.

    D. A milestone is a measurement of significant progress.

84. **The executive nurse heard the term *clinical systems analyst* and asks you to explain that term. What is the best response?**

    A. A clinical systems analyst manages the financial aspects of the clinical system.

    B. A clinical systems analyst identifies the clinical requirements of the clinical system and translates clinical requirements into clinical specifications for the system.

    C. A clinical systems analyst manages the clinical system project.

    D. A clinical systems analyst develops the systems from specifications provided by stakeholders and clinicians who are going to use the clinical system.

85. **During a meeting, the MIS director tells the executive nurse that an RFI is the next step in the process of the electronic medical records system. The executive nurse asks you to explain this term. What is the best response?**

    A. A request for proposal

    B. A proposal

    C. A request for information

    D. A request for instruction

86. **How is a primary key of a table used in a database?**

    A. A primary key uniquely identifies each instance of an attribute.

    B. A primary key uniquely identifies each instance of an entity.

    C. A primary key uniquely identifies all instances of an entity.

    D. A primary key uniquely identifies all instances of an attribute.

87. **The MIS director told the executive nurse that she was assembling a resource list. The executive nurse asks you to explain the concept of a resource list. What is the best response?**

    A. The resource list contains available resources, time available to work on the project, and costs associated with the resource.

    B. The resource list is a list of assignments for each resource working on the project.

    C. The resource list is used by the finance department to pay employees who work on the project.

    D. The resource lists contains the rationale for employing each resource on the project.

88. **What is meant by negotiable factors in planning for negotiations?**

    A. Negotiable factors are factors that will not stop the healthcare facility from agreeing with the vendor.

    B. Negotiable factors are factors that are nice to have but will not stop the healthcare facility from agreeing with the vendor.

    C. Negotiable factors are factors that must be in the agreement.

    D. Negotiable factors are factors agreed to with the vendor.

89. **What is a database access point?**

    A. A database access point is an entrance into the database that contains patient medical records.

    B. A database access point is an entrance into a computing device that contains patient medical records.

    C. A database access point is an entrance into computing device that displays patient medical records.

    D. A database access point is an entrance into an application that contains healthcare facility's records.

90. **The executive nurse asks you to explain the term *relationship capital*. What is the best response?**

    A. Relationship capital is the influence that the nursing informatics specialist has with the MIS department.

    B. Relationship capital is the influence that the nursing informatics specialist has with the vendor.

    C. Relationship capital is the ability to influence the project sponsor.

    D. Relationship capital is the reputation the nursing informatics specialist has with others in the healthcare facility that is used to build trust during a project.

91. **The executive nurse stated that the MIS director said a system was a multitasking system. What is the best explanation of multitasking?**

    A. Multitasking is a computer with a single central processor.

    B. Multitasking is when two or more tasks are performed by the computer at the same time.

    C. Multitasking is when two or more tasks seem to be performed by the computer at the same time.

    D. Multitasking is a computer with two central processors.

92. **During a planning meeting, the MIS director stated that all systems should be scalable. After the meeting, the executive asks you to explain this term. What is the best response?**

    A. It is the ability to increase and decrease in volume without having to reprogram the application.
    B. It is choosing the most appropriate staff for the project.
    C. It is recognizing that there is no one-size-fits-all application.
    D. It is balancing the application's benefits and deficits.

93. **Describe the concept of resource over allocation.**

    A. It is allocating too many resources to a task.
    B. It is allocating a resource to tasks beyond the time that the resource is available to work on the project.
    C. It is allocating a shared resource to the project.
    D. It is allocating stakeholders to tasks on the project.

94. **What is a recovery point objective?**

    A. A recovery point objective is the unacceptable period of time when a process can be available.
    B. A recovery point objective is the acceptable period of time when a process can be available.
    C. A recovery point objective is the unacceptable period of time when a process can be unavailable.
    D. A recovery point objective is the acceptable period of time when a process can be unavailable.

95. **What is the primary risk for identity theft for the healthcare facility?**

    A. Theft of a patient's visit number
    B. Theft of patient's credit card information
    C. A patient presenting another patient's medical benefits information when requesting medical care by the healthcare facility
    D. Thefts of a patient's medical records number

96. **The executive nurse asks you to explain the term** *bargaining range.* **What is your best response?**

    A. The difference between the healthcare facility's initial offer and the healthcare facility's final offer is the bargaining range.
    B. The difference between the healthcare facility's counter offer and the vendor's final offer is the bargaining range.
    C. The difference between the healthcare facility's initial offer and the vendor's counteroffer is the bargaining range.
    D. The difference between the healthcare facility's initial offer and the vendor's final offer is the bargaining range.

97. **What is meant by the term *breakpoint*?**

    A. Breakpoint is a cooling off period when both parties break from negotiations.
    B. Breakpoint is the best terms that are acceptable to the healthcare facility.
    C. Breakpoint is when the healthcare facility decides to settle with the vendor.
    D. Breakpoint is the least terms that are acceptable to the healthcare facility.

98. **A senior nurse is taking a course in nursing informatics and asks you the purpose of pseudo code. What is the best response?**

    A. Pseudo code decreases logical errors in the system.
    B. Pseudo code increases steps in the logical flow of a process.
    C. Pseudo code is a step-by-step description of the logical flow of a process.
    D. Pseudo code decreases steps in the logical flow of a process.

99. **During an interview for a nurse informatics position, the interviewer asks you to explain the concept of normalization. What is the best response?**

    A. Normalization is the process of removing duplicate data in a database design.
    B. Normalization is the process of duplicate data in a database design.
    C. Normalization is the process of developing indexes in a database design.
    D. Normalization is the process of balancing data in a database design.

100. **What is a business associate as defined by the Omnibus rule?**

    A. A business associate is any vendor used by the healthcare provider to manage patient medical records.
    B. A business associate is any vendor used by the healthcare provider to manage patient medical records. A business associate is required to comply with HIPAA regulations.
    C. A business associate is any employee who manages patient medical records. A business associate is required to comply with HIPAA regulations.
    D. A business associate is any employee who manages patient medical records.

FINAL EXAM ANSWERS

1. B. The TRANSACTION statement defines a group of SQL statements that form a transaction.
2. C. The wave's peak is considered a binary 1, and a wave's trough is considered a binary 0.
3. C. Negotiating in good faith means that a party is sincerely interested in reaching an agreement.
4. D. Data in motion is protected healthcare information that is being transmitted over a network.

5. B. Queries are embedded into programs or entered into an SQL console.
6. C. Information is processed as the information is received. The processing result is immediate.
7. D. Use Column Functions.
8. D. The person receiving the message may not be in the frame of mind to listen and understand the message.
9. A. A legacy system is a process that has not been reviewed or upgraded for a long time but provides an important process in the operations of the healthcare facility.
10. D. The emergency incident commander.
11. A. Cost of ownership is the total cost of acquiring and using a good or service.
12. C. Knowing what does not work is just as important as knowing what does work.
13. C. At the start of the project.
14. A. Distinct clause.
15. A. The number of clicks to perform a task to the minimum.
16. C. A system is a way of doing something to achieve a desired result.
17. D. Agile project methodology is used for relatively small, routine, less complex projects that can be accomplished by a team of up to nine members who are cross-functional.
18. D. Network broadcast.
19. B. A goal of an informatics security audit is to reduce the number of database access points.
20. C. A natural disaster is caused by an act of nature. A human-made disaster is caused by an unintentional or intentional act of a person.
21. C. The transfer of packets between networks.
22. C. Mediation is a process during which the mediator helps two sides find common ground.
23. D. Duration is the length of time resources work on a task plus elapsed time.
24. C. Data modeling is a method used to define data requirements of a clinical process and identify relationships between data elements.
25. C. A process of decomposing a simple request into smaller and smaller components that are easy to comprehend and analyze.
26. C. Meaningful use.
27. D. SQL is a type of programming language specifically designed to interact with DBMS to retrieve and manipulate information in the clinical database.
28. D. Understanding of group dynamics can help the nurse informatics project manager keep the project team and stakeholders focused on the project.
29. D. An arbitrator helps both parties settle a dispute.
30. B. Denial of service is a technique used to prevent access to a web server by sending very large numbers of requests to the web server, preventing others from accessing the web server.
31. D. A disaster recovery plan focuses on restoring operation during the first week of the disaster. A business continuity plan focuses on restoring operations after the first week of the disaster.

32. B. ASCII.
33. C. A sprint is a unit of work that last a fixed duration such as 1 week but can be upwards to 1 month.
34. C. Use the WHERE clause.
35. C. A foreign key is a foreign key of another table and is used to define a dependent relation.
36. D. A leveling diagram is a data flow diagram that gradually breaks down a process into details of the process.
37. D. A transaction processing system captures, processes, and stores information.
38. B. A database management system is a computer application that manages information stored in the database.
39. D. A task is an action that has a beginning and an end that produces a result.
40. D. To detect network traffic and collisions of packets.
41. C. Value is the perception of worth. The perception of value is used in negotiation to create a relatively low-cost incentive to reach the terms of a contract.
42. A. Risk tolerance is the amount of risk that the administrator is comfortable with accepting related to a risk associated with a disaster.
43. C. A digital certificate is a unique code issued by a known certificate authority certifying that a web server is trusted.
44. D. A progress payment is payment to the vendor for work completed during the project.
45. A. Two.
46. C. The RACI chart identifies responsibility and accountability and who has to be consulted and informed about the project.
47. D. A stored procedure is a query that resides on the DBMS and can be executed by calling the name of the stored procedure in an SQL statement.
48. A. An instance of an entity is data associated with the entity.
49. D. System owner.
50. D. It is a computer where applications are stored and distributed from when requested by users.
51. D. A database server is a computer connected to a network that enables computers throughout the healthcare facility to access the database.
52. B. A project charter specifies what the project manager is to deliver and the terms under which the project manager will manage the project.
53. C. A virtual team is a project team in which the participants join to complete a specific task and then leave the team after the task is completed.
54. D. Over- or understatement of work.
55. D. The data synchronization point is when data is backed up.
56. B. A key is a code used in a mathematical algorithm to encode and decode the information.
57. A. Accept, mitigate, transfer, and avoid.
58. C. A device connected to the network.

59. D. SBAR is a framework for communicating effectively so decisions can be made quickly.
60. B. Using a join.
61. A. In a relational database design, most duplicate information is removed from the database.
62. B. A stakeholder is any person who has an interest in an existing or proposed clinical information system.
63. A. Consultant, educator, researcher, and analyst.
64. D. A clinical database is the electronic repository of patient information or information necessary for patient care.
65. C. A stored procedure reduces the transmission time necessary to execute a query.
66. C. The stages of adoption is a process for adopting a proposal.
67. C. It is any device that can interact with a network.
68. D. A method is a behavior of an object.
69. B. A clinical information system is an arrangement of patients and the patients' medical teams, data, processes, and information technology that interact to collect, process, store, and provide as output the information needed to care for the patients.
70. B. Referential integrity occurs when a foreign key value matches a primary key value in a relation.
71. A. A naming convention standardizes how names of columns are written, making the names easy for the person writing or reading the query to read and identify the kind of information stored in the column.
72. C. The steering committee is a group of influential leaders who act as a sounding board for the nurse informatics specialist during the life of the project.
73. A. The healthcare facility will penalize the vendor 1% of the price for each month over the scheduled deadline.
74. D. A firewall is a filter between the healthcare facility's network and computing devices connected to the network and the outside world such as the Internet.
75. C. A service level of agreement is a contract that specifies the minimal level of service that a vendor will provide to the healthcare facility.
76. D. Emails remain on the local computer.
77. C. A physical database design contains technical specifications for storing data.
78. D. It ensures that all clinical systems are able to work together.
79. D. A personal health identifier is personal information about a patient that is designated as private and is protected under the HIPAA privacy rule.
80. B. Detective measures are processes that discovered that a disaster occurred.
81. D. An electronic envelop used to transmit information over the network.
82. A. The risk management plan identifies risks associated with project development and defines how the nurse informatics project manager will address each risk.
83. B. A milestone is a measurement of significant progress.
84. B. A clinical systems analyst identifies the clinical requirements of the clinical system and translates clinical requirements into clinical specifications for the system.

85. C. A request for information.
86. B. A primary key uniquely identifies each instance of an entity.
87. A. The resource list contains available resources, time available to work on the project, and costs associated with the resource.
88. B. Negotiable factors are factors that are nice to have but will not stop the health-care facility from agreeing with the vendor.
89. A. A database access point is an entrance into the database that contains patient medical records.
90. D. Relationship capital is the reputation the nurse informatics specialist has with others in the healthcare facility that is used to build trust during a project.
91. B. Multitasking is when two or more tasks are performed by the computer at the same time.
92. A. It is the ability to increase and decrease in volume without having to reprogram the application.
93. B. It is allocating a resource to tasks beyond the time that the resource is available to work on the project.
94. D. A recovery point objective is the acceptable period of time when a process can be unavailable.
95. C. A patient presenting another patient's medical benefits information when requesting medical care by the healthcare facility.
96. B. The difference between the healthcare facility's counteroffer and the vendor's final offer is the bargaining range.
97. D. Breakpoint is the least terms that are acceptable to the healthcare facility.
98. A. Pseudo code decreases logical errors in the system.
99. A. Normalization is the process of removing duplicate data in a database design.
100. B. A business associate is any vendor used by the healthcare provider to manage patient medical records. A business associate is required to comply with HIPAA regulations.

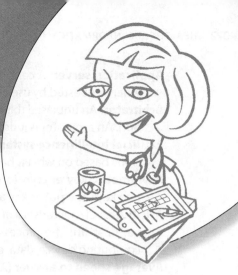

Glossary

Abandonment rate (ABA): The percentage of callers whose calls are not answered. The caller who is on a wait queue hangs up.

Acceptance: The action that clearly agrees to the offer. Acceptance can be conveyed in words, deeds, or performance in accordance with terms of the offer. Actions contrary to the offer can be construed as rejecting the offer or making a counteroffer. Acceptance must occur within a reasonable time.

Acceptance process: The way that the project sponsor and stakeholder verify that a project meets expectations and performs according to specifications.

Adaptive system: A system that can change based on the input.

Advanced Encryption Standard (AES): A high level encryption standard developed by the National Institute of Standards and Technology and adopted by the U.S. government.

Alias: An alternative name.

ALTER clause: Tells the DBMS that table or other object specified in the query is being modified.

American Recovery and Reinvestment Act: A federal law designed to help the economy recover from the 2008 financial crisis. Among its provision is billions of dollars to modernize health information technology systems.

American Standard Code for Information Interchange (ASCII): A coding standard that translates letters, numbers, and symbols to a number value.

Analog wave: Wave that is generated by alternating electrical current, causing the wave to fluctuate between above and below the baseline.

Application architecture: Technology used to implement the information systems. For example, a system might reside on a central computer called a server and referred to as clients by other computers.

Application server: A computer where applications are stored and distributed from when requested by users.

Arbitrator: An unbiased third party who resolves a dispute in a process called arbitration. An arbitrator is judge and jury.

Artificial intelligence system: A system that has the ability to learn and make decisions based on what it has learned.

Asymmetric key encryption: Commonly referred to as public key encryption. Uses two keys, the public key and the private key, to encode and decode information.

Attributes: Characteristics of an entity; information about an entity.

Authentication: The process of verifying that a person has permission to access a computing device, data, or a facility.

Average speed to answer (ASA): The number of seconds for the helpdesk to answer the phone.

Batch processing: When all information that needs processing is stored (called batching) and the batch is processed at the same time.

Behavior: A thing that the object can do (commonly referred to as a method, operation, or service).

Binary number system: A system that has two digits, 0 and 1. This is referred to as a base 2 numbering system.

Bluetooth: A protocol that enables computing devices and electronic devices to connect with each other using a low-powered radio frequency transmitter transmitting at 2.45 Ghz.

Breach of contract: Occurs when one party to a contract fails to perform some or all terms of the contract without legal cause.

Breakpoint: The least terms that are acceptable to the healthcare facility such as required factors.

Bridge: An electronic device that regenerates the signal similar to the actions of a repeater plus regulates network traffic enabling frames to be exchanged among segments.

Bus: The electronic pathway etched into the motherboard over which instructions and data flow to components.

Business associates: Vendors used by a healthcare provider to manage patient medical records. Business associates are required to comply with HIPAA regulations.

Business continuity plan: A plan that focuses on how to continue business operations during and following a disaster such as a power disruption.

Business impact analysis: Focuses on the impact a disaster has on the operations of the healthcare facility.

Business risk: Risk associated with doing business.

CamelCase: A naming convention using uppercase for the beginning of each word in a name.

Capacity: The ability to achieve a result such as the capacity to electronically store a million patient records.

Cardinality of relationships: The relationship between entities.

Carrier-sense multiple access: A protocol used to determine there is no traffic on the network before information is transmitted across the network.

Cascade delete rule: Rule stating that parent information and corresponding children information must be deleted automatically when the parent information is deleted.

Catastrophic event: A large-scale event that disrupts normal operations.

Central processing unit: The hardware device inside the computer that performs most processing of instructions.

Chain of command: A command hierarchy used to define a way in which orders are given and carried out within a group.

Change management: A process initiated at the beginning of a project to deal with changes in the project scope after the project is approved.

Change theory: Theory that focuses on implementing change from manual systems to technology-based systems within the healthcare environment.

CHECK clause: Used to limit the value range that can be placed in a column.

Chipset: Large-scale integrated circuits that make the motherboard come alive by coordinating the activities of the circuits and components that are integrated into the motherboard.

Classes of emergency: Defines the emergency condition by the length of time of the emergency.

Client/server architecture: A major improvement over file server architecture. The presentation layer and application layer are on the client. The data manipulation layer and the database are on the server.

Clinical computer network: The electronic highway over which clinical information travels among computers.

Clinical data reporting: Enables the nurse informatics specialist to interact with the clinical database directly to extract clinical information for reports.

Clinical database analysis: The process of transforming the data requirements of a clinical information system into a database design that efficiently stores clinical information for use by a clinical information application.

Clinical database application: A program or a group of programs used to store, retrieve, and manipulate clinical information such as a patient's medical record.

Clinical informatics team management: Enables the nurse informatics specialist to manage the project team, the clinical project sponsor, and the stakeholders throughout the project.

Clinical information system: An arrangement of patients and the patient's medical team, data, processes, and information technology that interact to collect, process, store, and provide as output the information needed to care for a patient.

Clinical project management: Enables the nurse informatics specialist to design a detailed plan on how to transform an idea into a working clinical information system.

Clinical project manager: Person responsible for planning, building, and delivering the completed project. The project manager is also responsible for managing the team and delivering the clinical system.

Clinical systems analysis: The process of analyzing the needs for a clinical system based on the workflow of the healthcare facility.

Clinical systems analyst: A person who identifies and translates clinical business flows into a set of instructions that form the basis of a clinical application.

Clinical systems designer: Person responsible for translating clinical specifications into technical specifications.

Clinical systems developer: Person responsible for building the clinical system based on technical specifications. A clinical systems developer may focus on a particular aspect of development such as databases, user interfaces, or back-end processing.

Closed system: A system that uses sensors as input and does not require humans.

Cloud architecture: A distribution architecture that makes files, applications, and the database available anytime from anywhere. This is an on-demand, broad network that can use any distributive architecture.

Cluster index: An index created from more than one column of a table in a database.

Cognitive theory: Theory that focuses on the input, output, and processing necessary to accomplish the goal of a system.

Collision detection CSMA/CD: A protocol used to detect if a packet of data interferes with another packet of data during transmission over an Ethernet network.

Column: A set of data values of a particular type in a table.

Comparison operators: An operator that compares expressions on both sides of the operator to determine if they are the same or different.

Compiler: A program that translates source code into the computer's native machine language.

Composite attribute: An attribute that has meaningful component parts.

Computer virus: A small, malicious program that attaches to a file or application program. The computer virus activates when the file is opened or the application program runs whatever disruption that the computer virus programmer intended. The virus may also attach itself to other files and applications.

Computerized physician order entry (CPOE): System that enables practitioners to enter orders directly into the computer. The CPOE system then transmits orders to the order management system for processing.

Computing device: Any device on the network that can send and receive information. Although many of these devices are computers, some are devices that normally are not recognized as a computer such as a printer that is directly connected to the network.

Configuration table: A collection of information with an associated network address used by a router to distribute packets of data over a network.

Consideration: Something of value promised to the party who makes the offer. The value can be money, a product, or a service.

Constraint: A restriction of information that can be stored in the database based on clinical rules. The constraint can be any logical statement that has a true or false result.

Contract: An agreement between two or more persons to do something or to refrain from doing something in exchange for something of value called consideration.

Corporation: A legal entity authorized by the government to act as person formed by individuals called stockholders.

Corrective measures: Processes that restore functionality to the healthcare facility during or after a disaster.

Cost estimates: The project manager's projected cost of a project.

Cost of ownership: The total cost of acquiring and using a good or service. This includes development, implementation, and maintenance.

Cost variance: The difference between budgeted and actual cost.

Critical path analysis: Analysis that determines tasks that will affect the duration of the project. That is, a change in the duration of tasks that fall on the critical path affects the duration of the project.

Customized application: An application that has been created to meet the specific needs of the healthcare facility. The customized application mimics the healthcare facility's manual process, requiring minimum training and change in the work flow.

Cyclic redundancy check (CRC): An error detecting code used to determine if packets of data were received intact over a network or from a storage device.

Data at rest: Protected healthcare information stored on a server or other computing device.

Data capture: The identification and acquisition of new data at the source of the data, which is usually data entry but also can be electronic data transferred from another computing device.

Data control language (DCL): Consists of commands that control database functions.

Data definition language (DDL): Consists of commands used to define a database and tables.

Data disposed: Protected healthcare information that is being destroyed.

Data encryption standard (DES): An encryption method that uses a private key to encrypt data.

Data entry: The process of translating source data into a computer readable format; occurs by using a data input device such as a keyboard, a mouse, touch screens, a bar code reader, smart cards, or a biometric reader.

Data: A distinct piece of information.

Data flow diagram: Also known as a context diagram; used to analyze a work package. A data flow diagram is an illustration of a workflow.

Data in motion: Protected healthcare information that is being transmitted over a network. Data can be encrypted at the network layer of the OSI model using commercially available encryption software.

Data in use: Protected healthcare information that is being created, retrieved, updated, or deleted. Privacy screens on monitors and restricted positions of monitors away from public view are the best methods to protect data being used by staff.

Data manipulation language (DML): Consists of commands used to maintain the database and to query a database.

Data modeling: A method used to define data requirements of a clinical process and identify relationships between data elements.

Data recovery: The process of restoring data after an event that disabled the database.

Data synchronization point: The point at which data is backed up. Depending on the design of the application, data can be backed up either immediately after a transaction or on a schedule.

Database: An electronic filing cabinet that contains clinical information.

Database access points: An entrance into the database that contains patient medical records.

Database backup: A copy of the database that is copied to the primary database to restore the database to a state before the database failure.

Database index: Similar to an index of a book in that the index contains the data being searched and the location of that data in the table.

Database management system (DBMS): A computer application that manages information stored in the database.

Database server: A computer that runs a database management system.

Database system: A system that stores and retrieves data and is usually integrated with other types of system.

Decision support system: A system that assists the manager in making decisions by analyzing information stored in a database.

Deliverables: The result of performing a task.

Demilitarized zone (DMZ): A physical or logical portion of an organization's network that is exposed to untrusted network outside the organization such as the Internet.

Denial of service: A technique used by an unscrupulous person or group to prevent access to a computing device, typically a web server.

Dependencies: A task that cannot begin until another task is completed.

Derived attribute: A value that can be calculated from related attribute values.

Detection risk: A risk that occurs because the clinical project manager or an advisor uses faulty procedures or bases a decision on unknowingly false information.

Detective measures: Processes that discover that a disaster occurred. For example, activation of a fire alarm signals a fire is a detective measure common to all healthcare facilities.

Development: The effort to get an item ready to use.

Digital: Discrete values are used to represent data.

Digital certificates: A unique code issued by a known certificate authority certifying that a web server is trusted. That is, the web server is who it says it is.

Digital wave: A wave that consists of positive voltage. That is, the height of the wave is present (the value one) or not present (the value zero).

Direct impact: An event or task that affects another event or task without any intermediate operations.

Disabling services: The act of making a service unavailable.

Disaster: A catastrophic event that may cause significant damage and the possible loss of life.

Disaster drills: A practice response to a potential disaster in the absence of the disaster.

Disaster recovery: The process of restoring function to the healthcare facility during and after the disaster.

Disaster recovery plan: A plan that focuses on returning the healthcare facility to marginal functionality within the first week of a disaster.

Disincentives: Things of value to the healthcare facility—and not to the vendor—that should occur if certain actions do not occur.

DISTINCT clause: The clause removes duplicate data from the result set specified in the SELECT clause.

Downtime procedures: Processes that are enacted when a disaster or emergency occurs.

DROP statement: Removal of an object such as a table or database that is specified in the DROP statement.

Duration: The length of time resources work on a task plus elapsed time.

E-commerce system: A system used to conduct business over the Internet.

Effective listening: The use of multiple senses to understand the spoken message.

Electromagnetic spectrum: The range of all possible frequencies of electronmagnetic radiation.

Electronic health record: System that enables the staff to enter, store, and retrieve a patient's medical record using a computer system.

Electronic medication administration record: System that enables staff to enter, store, and retrieve medication orders and document medication administration. The system also interacts with the electronic pharmacy system to track inventory and billing for medications.

Elements of a contract: Portions of an agreement necessary for the agreement to be considered a legal contract.

Emergency operations center (EOC): A location in the healthcare facility where a disaster is managed. Typically, the EOC is located in a central location within the facility such as a large conference room or auditorium.

Employee: A person who performs an action for wages or salary paid by another person or organization called an employer under work terms specified by the employer.

Encryption: The process of scrambling information called encoding so the information is not readable without deciphering.

Entities: People, places, things, or events.

Entity attribute: A characteristic of an entity such as a person's name.

Entity instance: Information about an entity.

Entity relationships: The association between two or more entities such as a patient having many medication orders.

Entity type: A collection of entity instances such as patients.

Executable program: A program that is loaded onto a computer and loaded into memory when a user wants to run the application.

Expert system: A system designed to provide advice that would otherwise be offered by an expert.

Fact finder: An unbiased third party whose sole purpose is to review relevant information, including contracts, performance records, industry standards, and other elements that influence the dispute. The fact finder assembles facts into a logical flow and presents a list of facts to both parties.

Feedback: An adjustment to the input based on the output such as taking another blood sample if the blood glucose level is unusual.

File server: A computer that enables multiple users to save and use files to the same disk. This is similar to a shared hard disk.

File server architecture: A computer that stores and serves up files.

Financially solvent: Able to meet financial obligations.

Firewall: A filter between the healthcare facility's network and computing devices connected to the network and the outside world such as the Internet. A firewall can be a computer program that filters all communication coming from the Internet and going to the Internet from computing devices on the network. A firewall might also be a detected computing device that filters communication based on rules established by the healthcare facility.

First call resolution (FCR): A percentage of calls to a helpdesk that are resolved without the callers calling the helpdesk again.

First normal form: Rearrange information so each column in a table contains one value and there are no duplicate values.

FOR clause: Used to specify the table name following the ALIAS clause.

Frame: A digital data transmission unit.

FUD factor: Fear, uncertainty, or doubt of continuity that can lead to a disaster.

Gantt chart: A visual depiction of the work plan.

General contractor: A vendor that takes on responsibility for the entire project and engages specialty contractors to complete their portions of the contract.

General partnership: A partnership in which each partner is responsible for the liability of the partnership. That is, a general partner's personal assets can be used by creditors to pay the liabilities of the partnership.

Gift: To transfer something of value without receiving something (consideration) in return for the transfer.

Goods: Material that is in demand by another person.

GRANT clause: Assigns rights to access the database or a portion of the database.

GROUP BY clause: Aggregates results of a SELECT clause.

HAVING clause: Combined with the GROUP BY clause to restrict groups of rows returned by a query.

Health Information Technology for Economic and Clinical Health (HITECH) Act: Federal law that stimulates adoption of electronic health records.

Health Insurance Portability and Accountability Act (HIPAA): Federal law that provides rights and protection for personal health information.

Hospital Emergency Incident Command System (HEICS): The system that takes over operations of a healthcare facility during a disaster or emergency.

Human-made disaster: An act of humans such as failure of the infrastructure or a hazardous material spill. A human-made disaster may be preventable by monitoring and implementing procedures that reduce the likelihood of such an event.

Hypertext Transfer Protocol (HTTP): A protocol for distribution of collaborative information over the web.

Identity theft: Commonly referred to identity fraud; the process of acquiring identification of another person and using the identification to impersonate that person.

Incentive: Something of value to the vendor that can be offered if the vendor performs certain actions.

Index: A list of keywords and reference to keyword locations in a database.

Indirect impact: An event or task that affects another event or task with an intermediate operation.

Individual: A legal entity that can conduct business. The individual pays all expenses associated with the business and receives all revenues generated by the business. The individual is also personally liable to fulfill obligations stated in a contract with a customer. The individual manages the business.

Industry standards: An agreed upon specification by members of an industry.

Information disclosure: Revealing information.

Inherent risk: A natural risk that exists in any project. For example, key employees are unable to work because of illness.

Input: The activity of gathering data such as a blood sample.

Input devices: A mechanism for entering information into a computer.

Installation test: The final test of the system before the organization uses the system. The installation test occurs immediately after the system is installed in the production environment and before the system goes live. The goal is to uncover any problems that may prevent the organization from using the system.

Integrated systems: A network of systems that interact with each other to provide nearly seamless processing.

Integration test: A test of all components of the system to determine if components work well together. This testing is usually performed in the test environment.

Inter-company systems: Systems that are able to share data between two independent organizations.

Internet: A global network of networks connected by powerful routers operated by telecommunication companies using the TCP/IP protocols.

Internet Mail Access Protocol server (IMAP): A protocol enabling a client to access and manipulate email on a server.

Intranet: A private network typically within an organization; it works on the same basic principles as the Internet.

Job action sheet: Sheet that lists each position in the command structure and the corresponding roles and responsibilities.

Key: A code used in a mathematical algorithm to encode and decode information.

Left outer join: Links two tables by returning rows of the left table in the WHERE clause that matches the left table and does not match the right table. Only rows in the right table that match the left table are returned.

Legacy system: A process critical to the operations of the healthcare facility that has not been reviewed or upgraded for a long time. A legacy system can be a computer-based system, a manual system, or a combination.

Legal entity: An organization, such as a vendor, that has the right to act as a person.

Leveling diagram: A form of a data flow diagram at a level of detail in the process. Leveling diagrams are used to discuss the clinical process with stakeholders, each of whom may have a different view of the process.

Liability: Legal responsibility for something.

License: A right to use an application under specific terms of the license. A license can be granted on a per computer basis using the application based on the full-time equivalent clinical employees at the healthcare facility or by the number of con-current users.

Limited liability partnership: A partnership that legally limits a partner's liability to the partner's investment in the partnership. The limited liability partner's personal assets cannot be used by creditors to pay the liability of the partnership. Each partner participates in managing the business based on the partnership agreement. The partnership agreement specifies terms of the partnership. That is, one partner may manage the business (managing partner), and other partners are advisors. Alternatively, all partners manage the business.

Local application architecture: Architecture in which all three components reside on the same computer.

Local area network (LAN): Network technology that connects computing devices that are relatively close to each other such as in the same healthcare facility.

Logical database design: Defines relationships among entities.

Mail server: A computer that stores emails that contains an application that runs the email service for the organization.

Management clinical information technology: The application of computer technology and management information systems to the clinical setting.

Management information systems: A system designed to provide information to assist managers to make decisions.

Mapping: The process of transforming a logical database design to a physical database design. The goal of mapping is to identify and define fields of data commonly referred to as a column.

Material breach: A breach that occurs when one party receives something substantially different than that specified in the contract. For example, a material breach occurs if the electronic medical records system does not perform as specified in the contract.

Meaningful use: A mandate by the federal government to use electronic applications to improve quality, safety, communication, and coordination of healthcare.

Media access control (MAC): The permanent address of a computing device that is assigned by the device manufacturer.

Mediation: A third party who attempts to bring together two disagreeing parties.

Mediator: An unbiased third party who is trained to mediate disputes. The goal of a mediator is to help both parties to resolve a conflict.

Method: A set of instructions that performs a function.

Migration plan: A plan that moves the system into the production environment.

Milestones: A measurement of significant progress.

Minor breach: A breach that occurs when the other party receives substantial things—but not everything—specified in the contract.

Motherboard: The largest circuit board inside the computer that contains many components, two of which are memory chips and the processor.

Multitasking: Performing more than one task simultaneously.

Multi-user: An operating system that enables many users access to the computer at the same time and is used on mainframe computers and shared computers called servers.

Mutuality: Both parties to the contract understand the terms of the contract when the contract is signed.

Natural disasters: Acts of nature such as storms, floods, and earthquakes. Natural disasters cannot be prevented.

Negotiable factors: Factors that are nice to have but will not stop the healthcare facility from agreeing with the vendor.

Negotiation: The process of two or more parties reaching an agreement.

Negotiation strategy: An action plan used to reach an agreement with another party.

Network server: A computer that manages the computer network. It grants permission to use the network and routes network traffic to the desired destination.

Network: Interconnection of computing devices.

Nonadaptive system: A system that is unable to change based on input.

Normalization: The process of removing duplicate data.

Not required factors: Factors that are unimportant to the healthcare facility.

Nursing informatics: The area of nursing that combines nursing, information, and computer sciences to manage information required for use in the nursing practice. The American Nurses Association defines nursing informatics as a specialty that integrates nursing science, computer science, and information science to manage and communicate data, information, knowledge, and wisdom in nursing practice.

Object: Very similar to an entity because both have attributes. However, an object also has behaviors.

Object-oriented design: Design that uses a natural approach to designing a clinical system.

Offer: The promise to act or refrain from doing something some time in the future.

Office automation system: A system designed to improve common activities in the office, including word processing, spreadsheets, email, and other programs typically purchased from a vendor.

Off-the-shelf application: An application purchased from a vendor; the application cannot be modified by the healthcare facility. The healthcare facility is likely required to adopt the workflow built into the vendor's application.

Omnibus rule: The HIPAA rule that increases patient privacy and security of patient medical records.

OODA loop models: Models used to support rapid planning by defining four stages in the decision process.

Open source: An application that is built by an open source initiative in which volunteers develop a portion of the application. Anyone can download and use the application free of charge as long as they abide by the open software foundation license that, among other limitations, states that they cannot charge for components of the open source application.

Open system: A system that requires human input. Most nursing informatics systems are open systems.

Open systems interconnection (OSI) model: A model that defines steps used to transmit information from a computing device over a network.

Operating systems: A collection of software that manages computer hardware.

Operational level of agreement: Similar in concept to the service level of agreement except the agreement is between internal entities within the healthcare facility.

Operational risk: Happens when the business logic is faulty, resulting in unexpected outcomes from the project.

Oral contract: A verbal agreement between two parties that contains all the elements of a contract. Although terms of the agreement are not written, the contract is enforceable under the law. However, the Statute of Fraud specifies that some contracts such as for real estate must be written.

Order management: System that enables staff to enter, store, and retrieve medical and nonmedical orders. In addition, the order management system interacts with other systems to receive and process orders.

Outer join: Returns rows of two tables whether or not values in the rows match.

Output: The production of useful information such as the blood glucose level in the sample of blood.

Outsourcing: Contracting out a business process to a third party.

Packets: Small pieces of information transmitted over a network.

Packet filtering: Inspection by firewall software of the content of data packet transmitted over a computer network.

Packet switching: A method of sending data packets over large networks.

Packet-switching network: A network designed with redundancy that uses a technique called load balancing to ensure packets reach their destination within an acceptable time period, typically measured in milliseconds. If a delay is detected during equipment malfunction, the packet-switching network automatically reroutes the packet to a different circuit.

Partnership: A legal entity formed by two or more individuals who work toward a common goal such as providing a product or service to earn a profit. Each partner provides value to the partnership in the form of assets (money or property). Partners then share the revenues and profits realized by the partnership.

Patient profile: Profile that consists of a standard set of information that is maintained for every patient that can be exchanged with and updated by any healthcare provider who is caring for the patient.

Patient Protection and Affordable Care Act: A federal law established to increase the quality and affordability of health insurance. Commonly called Obamacare.

Pattern matching: A method of comparing values with an expression.

Payment schedule: Times in the future when payment will be made.

Penalty clause: A provision in a contract that states consequences for failure to perform terms of the contract.

Performance incentive: A provision in a contract that states consideration above expected consideration if a party to the contract provides a service within special parameters stated in the contract.

Person: A legal entity such as an individual, partnership, or corporation.

Phase: Delivering a discrete product such as implementing an eMAR to acute units of a healthcare facility.

Physical access: The ability for people to gain access to a computer system.

Physical database design: Design that contains technical specifications for storing data.

Point of failure: An element in the healthcare facility's operation that might fail such as failure of the local area network from transmitting electronic data throughout the facility.

Point of presence: An access point to the Internet.

Post Office Server (POP3): A computer server that collects and maintains messages for each e-mail account using the Post Office Protocol.

Preventive measures: Processes that prevent a disaster from occurring. For example, placing power lines underground prevents loss of power from a storm disrupting power lines.

Primary key: A unique way to identify each instance of an entity such as a medical record number.

Primary storage: Main area of computer memory used to store information that is retrieved quickly by the central processing unit.

Print server: A computer that manages printing documents on printers that are located on the network. When print is selected by a user, the document is sent to the print server. Software on the print server sends the document to the designated printer.

Processing: The activity of transforming data into a useful output such as a glucose meter measuring a blood sample.

Processing method: The way processing occurs.

Procurement: The process of acquiring goods and services from one or more vendors. The goal is to make the acquisition at the best possible cost of ownership at the right quality, quantity, place, and time and from the right vendor.

Program: Contains explicit instructions to the central processing unit on what to do and when to do it.

Programmer: A member of the project team who is responsible for translating specifications and the design requirements into a program.

Progress payment: A portion of the total payment that the healthcare facility makes to the vendor at specific milestones during the project. The remaining payment is made when the healthcare facility accepts the delivered project. Progress payments help the vendor's cash flow during the project. Cash flow is the amount of funds paid and received. A progress payment replenishes funds that were expensed for a segment of the project.

Project: A temporary set of task performed to produce a desired outcome.

Project charter: A document that specifies what the project manager is to deliver and the terms under which the project manager will manage the project.

Project closure stage: The stage that begins after the project is fully developed and has passed all tests.

Project execution stage: The stage when the project team comes together to make the project sponsor's idea reality by following the project plan developed by the project manager.

Project initiation stage: The stage when the project sponsor identifies the clinical need for the project and develops a clinical case for launching the project.

Project life cycle: Phases of a project.

Project manager: The manager of the project and the project team. The project manager is also the facilitator of the project who coordinates project activities with the project sponsor and stakeholders and the project team to ensure that expectations are well defined and objectively measurable and that the project team delivers a system that meets the expectations of the project sponsor and stakeholders.

Project phase: A segment of the project life cycle.

Project planning stage: The stage when the project manager takes over the project and translates the project sponsor's idea into reality.

Project sponsor: The person within the healthcare facility who proposes the project to the administration and receives authorization to undertake the project.

Proposal: A formal document submitted by a vendor that specifies how the vendor intends to meet specifications in the request for proposal.

Protected health identifiers (PHIs): HIPAA-designated elements of patients' medical records that are considered protected health information.

Protocols: Agreed upon ways of doing things.

Proxy server: An intermediary between the computing device within the healthcare facility's access to the Internet and the website itself. The computing device never directly interacts with the Internet.

Pseudo code: A step-by-step description of the logical flow of a process.

Public key: An encryption method that uses a combination of a private key and public key. The public key is available to any computing device that wants to encrypt messages to a computer. The private key is used by the computer to decipher the encrypted message.

Quality assurance test: A test that determines if the system meets the standards of quality established by the organization. Typically, an internal group of quality testers or a vendor tries all possible scenarios for using the system, including scenarios that are unlikely to occur, with the goal of finding faults in the logic of the system. A quality assurance test is performed in the test environment.

Query: A request written using Structure Query Language (SQL) sent to a database management system (DBMS) to perform specific tasks.

RACI chart: Responsibility assignment matrix used to assign tasks. RACI stands for responsible, accountable, consulted, informed.

Rapid planning: A method used to adapt to dynamic and fast-changing situations.

Real-time planning: A technique for modifying plans based on the current situation.

Real-time operating system (RTOS): A system used to control machinery that has a skimpy user interface that enables the user to interact with the machine.

Real-time processing: Sometimes referred to as transactional processing; where information is processed as the information is received. The processing result is immediate.

Recovery point objective: The acceptable period of time when a process can be unavailable.

Recovery time objective: The time needed by management information systems to restore the process when a failure occurs.

Referential integrity: Occurs when a foreign key value matches a primary key value in a relation. For example, the patient's medical record number and visit identifier in the order table, which is a foreign key, match a patient's medical records number and visit identifier in the patient information table.

Regression test: A test performed when a defect occurs after a major change in the system is implemented that results in lost functionality. Typically, the regression test is conducted in the test environment.

Regulatory compliance: A process of adhering to rules established by regulatory authorities.

Relational database: Database design in which most duplicate information is removed from the database. The single instance of the data is placed in a table within the database and is referenced each time that information is needed.

Relationship capital: The reputation with colleagues that establishes credibility and trust.

Remote login: A login that enables a computing device called a host to take control over a remote computing device that is connected to the network.

Request for information: A formal document distributed to vendors asking each vendor to submit a response to questions contained in the document.

Request for proposal: A formal document distributed to vendors asking each vendor to submit a proposal for delivering the new clinical system.

Required factors: Factors that are not negotiable. If these factors are not in the final agreement, then there is no agreement, and the healthcare facility will walk away from negotiations.

Residual risk: A risk that remains after the clinical project manager has mitigated other risks.

Resource allocation: The process of assigning resources to tasks.

Resource: A thing or person required to complete a task or subtask.

Resource list: A list that contains a resource by title, the availability of the resource to the project, and the cost of the resource.

Restrict delete rule: A rule stating that no parent side information in a parent table (row) can be deleted unless all corresponding rows in children tables are also deleted. For example, if patient is removed from the patient information table, then all orders for the patient's medical records number and visit identifiers must also be removed.

Right outer join: Occurs when only rows in the left table that match rows in the right table in the WHERE clause are returned along with all the rows in the right table.

Risk: The possibility of harm or long-term loss as a result of an event.

Risk assessment: A process of assessing the magnitude of the potential loss related to interruption of operations such a disaster.

Risk responses: A strategy that defines actions to take to address exposure to danger of experience a loss.

Risk tolerance: The amount of risk administrators will tolerate.

Risks of procurement: Exposure to loss during the procurement process.

Rootkit: A stealth program that is difficult to detect because the rootkit modifies programs designed to detect computer viruses. A rootkit is a computer virus that modifies administrative tools used to manage the operations of a computing device and causes the administrative tool to make inappropriate decisions.

Router: An electronic device that logically divides a network into segments. A router uses rules (protocols) that are different than Ethernet. This means that a router can connect a variety of network technologies.

Row: A set of related data in a table.

Runtime library: A portion of an executable program that is added at the time when the program is executed. Runtime libraries enable programmers to change and distribute a portion of the application without having to compile the complete application and distribute a large executable program.

SBAR: A communication framework developed by the military in World War II to focus leaders on information needed to make decisions quickly. SBAR means situation, background, assessment, and recommendation.

Scalability: The ability to increase or decrease a clinical application to match changes in demand.

Scope statement: A brief expression of what will be delivered.

Second normal form: A primary key must identify groups of nonkey attributes for data to be in the second normal form. For example, all attributes of a patient are identified by a medical record number and visit identifier in a row of a table.

Secondary storage: Data storage outside the computer's primary (memory) storage such as a disk drive.

Secure Socket Link (SSL): Standard security technology used to establish an encrypted link between a server and client.

Security audit: A process of reviewing the healthcare facility to identify security risks such as access to the facility. A component of the security audit is to review electronic and manual processes involved in recording, storing, and retrieving medical records.

Server: A computer that is shared by many users over a computer network.

Service level of agreement (SLA): Contains objective metrics that both the vendor and the healthcare facility can use to measure the vendor's performance.

Shared values: Fundamental beliefs of group that guide the group's actions.

Simple Mail Transfer Protocol (SMTP): An Internet standard for transmission of electronic mail.

Single-user, multitasking: The most commonly used operating systems on personal computers.

Single-user, single task: Designed to enable one person to do one thing at a time.

Specifications: Define specifically what the computer application is to do.

SQL console: A software application used to send interactive SQL statements to a database management system (DBMS).

Stages of adoption: The evaluation process a person follows before adopting to change.

Stakeholder: An individual who has an interest in a process.

Stateful inspection: A firewall architecture that examines all parts of a packet when traversing a firewall.

Steering committee: The sounding board for a nurse informatics specialist, who can present issues and proposed solutions so the steering committee can assess the importance of the issue and practicality of the solution. The steering committee monitors key project metrics to determine if the project is on track.

Stored procedure: A query located at the database executed when the database management system (DBMS) receives a request from a client to execute the query.

Stress test: Test that determines how the system will perform under a higher than expected volume of transactions. Some clinical project managers believe that the stress test determines at what point the system will stop functioning. The stress test is performed in the test environment.

Structured data: Data stored in a fixed column within a row.

Structured Query Language (SQL): A programming language used to query a database management system (DBMS).

Subnet: A segment of a large network. All subnets are connected by a router.

Subquery: A query within a query.

Subtask: An action that has a beginning and an end and produces a result that is used as an action of another task.

Switch: A network device that forwards packets across networks.

Symmetric key encryption: Requires that the computing device receiving the encrypted information use the same key as the computing device that sends the encrypted information. A drawback of using symmetric key encryption is that computing devices receiving the encoded information must be known to the sender.

System: A way of doing something to achieve a desired result. A system can be a manual process such as driving to work, an electronic process such as documenting an admissions assessment in an electronic medical record, or a combination such as measuring blood glucose from a finger stick. A system has four elements: input, processing, output, and feedback.

System owner: An individual who is responsible for a system.

System test: One of the final tests performed before a system is placed in the production environment. The goal of the systems test is to determine if the system works well with other systems in the organization. The system test occurs in the staging environment. All systems except for the system being tested are systems currently running in the organization.

System user: An individual who uses a system.

Systems theory: Theory that focuses on the interactions between the use of technology and systems of the human body.

Table: An organized set of data elements in columns and rows.

Tailored application: An application that is purchased from a vendor that can be tailored to fit the workflow of the healthcare facility. The application is divided into two components, the core and modifiable components. The core component contains the processing logic of the application, and the modifiable component contains elements that can be changed by the healthcare facility, which is typically nomenclature, screens, and limited processing such as required information. The healthcare facility will likely adjust some but not necessarily all workflows to accommodate the application.

Task: An action that has a beginning and an end that produces a result.

TCP/IP: A standard for transmitting data over the Internet.

Team-driven planning: A group determines the directions of the group.

Technological risk: The chance that a key system will fail such as the infrastructure being unable to handle a data load.

Thin client: A computer (client) that depends heavily on another computer (server) to function.

Third normal form: The primary key must not be determined by another attribute of a table for the table to be in the third normal form.

Tiers: Distinct levels of a network to computer environment architecture.

Tier 1 carrier: An Internet Service Provider (e.g., Verizon, AT&T, Sprint) that has access to a region (e.g., country) of the Internet.

Tier system: A network or computer environment architecture that has distinct levels.

Time service factor (TSF): A percentage of calls that are answered within a specific time period.

Transaction: An activity that has a beginning, processing, and an end.

Transaction processing system: A system that captures, processes, and stores information. A patient admissions system is a transaction processing system because the system is used to collect, process, and store patient information.

Transport layer security (TLS): A protocol for security transmission of data over the Internet.

Trigger: An event that occurs in the database to cause the database management system (DBMS) to execute a stored procedure.

Trojan horse: A type of malware embedded in another program that activates when the program executes.

Turnaround time (TAT): The time necessary to complete a specific task.

Unauthorized access: Accessing a database or a computer without permission.

Unicode: A standard of representing text used in most of the world's writing system as a numeric value. Unicode-4 is used for the additional symbols. Unicode-4 uses a 32-bit (four bytes) number, which can handle about 1 million symbols. The most commonly used symbols in every language are assigned a Unicode-2 number. Therefore, most of the textual information is stored using 2 bytes per symbol. Unicode-4 symbols are inserted where necessary into the information.

Uniform Commercial Code: Standard laws for conducting commerce.

Uniform Resource Locator (URL): A protocol to locate resources on the World Wide Web.

Unit test: Sometimes referred to as a component test, it determines if a functional piece of the system meets specifications. Unit tests are conducted in either the development or test environments.

Unseen fail point: An unanticipated portion of a system that can malfunction.

Unstructured data: Data that is not organized.

Uptime (UT): The amount of time that the application, computing device, or data center is functioning. For example, a computing device maybe unavailable for 4 hours a week while the management information systems department performs maintenance on the device.

User acceptance test: Test that determines if the system is acceptable to the project sponsor and stakeholder and is an element of the acceptance process. The user acceptance test occurs in the test environment.

User interface: A computer program that enables clinicians to store, retrieve, edit, and delete clinical information.

Value: The perception of worth.

VALUES clause: Identifies values in an SQL query that are to be inserted into a table of a database.

Vendor: A person or organization that provides goods or services.

View: A virtual organization of data from two or more tables in a database.

Virtual project teams: A group that forms for a particular task and disbands after the task is completed.

Wave: Oscillation of matter through space accompanied by a transfer of energy.

Web-based application: A browser-based program accessible only on the Internet or intranet.

Web server: A computing device that stores websites and files associated with the website such as video and pictures. It is a computer that manages the organization's intranet (within the organization) and Internet (outside the organization).

Wide area network (WAN): Network technology that connects a smaller number of computing devices over a larger area such as connecting two or more healthcare facilities together.

Wi-Fi: A wireless network that uses radio waves to connect a computing device to the network.

Work breakdown structure: The process of decomposing a simple request into smaller and smaller components that are easy to comprehend and analyze.

Work group: A subset of the team that has a clear, measurable objective that addresses a portion of the project's objective. The work group has a work group leader who takes on many of the project manager's roles and responsibilities related to the work group. The work group is mutually accountable for achieving the work group's goal.

Work plan: A detailed description and organization of tasks and resources that are necessary to complete a project.

Worms: Malware that replicates itself and spreads to other computers.

Written contract: A document that contains term of an agreement between two parties. Contracts between the healthcare facility and vendors are typically written contracts.

Zero sum game: A competition that results in a winner and loser.

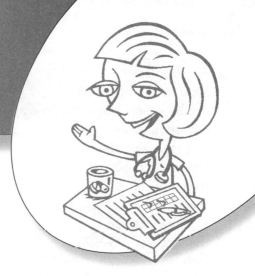

Index

Page numbers followed by *f* denote figures; those followed by *t* denote tables.

A

ABA. *See* abandonment rate
abacus, 9
abandonment rate, 254
acceptance
   of contract, 227
   of project, 132–133
   of risk, 130, 251
accountability, of stakeholders,
    152
act of God, 230
adaptive system, 30
administrator passwords, 269
administrators, 206
adoption, stages of, 224–225
advanced encryption standard, 278
Advanced Research Project Agency
    Network, 10
AES. *See* advanced encryption standard
aggressor, 150
agile project management
   backlog grooming, 138
   daily scrum, 138
   definition of, 135

focus board, 136, 136*f*
methodology of, 135–136
project team, 138–139
scrum approach to, 137–138
sprint, 137–138
agreement(s)
   operational level of, 255
   service-level, 234, 253–255
   of understanding, 221
alias, 83, 95
all-at-once migration strategy, 134
allocation of resources, 122–123, 123*f*
ALTER clause, 83
American Nurses Association, 2
American Recovery and Reinvestment Act,
    4–5
American Standard Code for Information
    Interchange, 175
analog waves, 176–178, 177*f*
AND operator, 87
API. *See* application programming
    interface
APIPA. *See* automatic private IP
    addressing

subtask, 115
task, 115–116
work package, 113
work groups, 144–145
working the contract, 231–234
work plan, 110
work rules, 1454
World Wide Web, 10, 192
worms, 287

WPA2. *See* Wi-Fi protected access
version 2
written communication, 154, 156
written contract, 226
WWW. *See* World Wide Web

Z

zero sum game, 214
zero value, 49